Primetime Pregnancy

Primetime Pregnancy

The Proven Program for Staying in Shape
Before and After Your Baby Is Born

Kathy Kaehler,
***Today* Show Fitness Consultant,**
and Cynthia Tivers

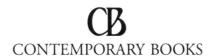

CONTEMPORARY BOOKS

Library of Congress Cataloging-in-Publication Data

Tivers, Cynthia.
    Primetime Pregnancy : the proven program for staying in shape
before and after your baby is born / Cynthia Tivers and Kathy
Kaehler.
       p.   cm.
    ISBN 0-8092-3072-0
    1. Exercise for pregnant women.   2. Physical fitness for
women.   3. Postnatal care.   I. Kaehler, Kathy.   II. Title.
RG558.7.T58   1997
618.2'4—dc21   97-29942
                                                   CIP

Cover design by Kim Bartko
Photo on p. xx by Dana Fineman
Cover photo and all other interior photos © David Roth
Interior design by Monica Baziuk

Published by Contemporary Books
An imprint of NTC/Contemporary Publishing Company
4255 West Touhy Avenue, Lincolnwood (Chicago), Illinois 60646-1975 U.S.A.
Copyright © 1998 by Kathy Kaehler and Cynthia Tivers
Printed in the United States of America
International Standard Book Number: 0-8092-3072-0

18   17   16   15   14   13   12   11   10   9   8   7   6   5   4   3   2

To me and my journey toward getting
my own body back
Kathy Kaehler

To a partner whose body, mind, and attitude
are inspirational
Cynthia Tivers

Contents

Acknowledgments

There are many people who helped give birth to this book and to whom we want to give thanks. First, of course, there are Cooper and Payton Koch, Kathy's and Billy's beautiful twin boys. We want to thank our editor Kara Leverte, whose never-ending patience and encouragement helped nurture this project from beginning to end; Stan Corwin, our wonderful agent and cheerleader; David Roth, whose photography makes this book so inviting; Deborah Schwartz, David's assistant extraordinaire; and our makeup artist, Cathy Highland, the lady with the deft touch. We want to give Noreen Green and her then-unborn baby, Aaron Michael, special thanks for posing for our pregnancy photos. We also want to thank Michelle Pfeiffer, Jami Gertz, Rita Wilson Hanks, Harriet Posner, Sheryl Berkoff Lowe, and Meg Ryan for generously sharing their pregnancy stories with us.

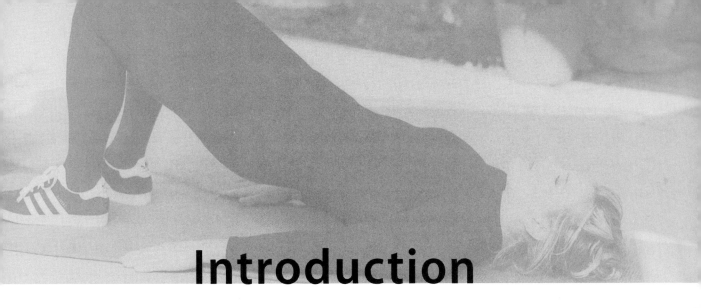

Introduction

It was Christmastime 1995 when Kathy, her husband, Billy, and their three Labs—Clyde, Bear, and Moose—stopped by to drop off a gift for me. Kathy and Billy looked happy and relaxed, glad that the holidays would give Kathy a break from a very hectic schedule. Within a six-month period, Kathy had completed four exercise videos with Claudia Schiffer (all shot overseas) and exercise videos for Reebok and for CBS Fox, and she and I had completed our first book, *Primetime Bodies*. In between, she was traveling back and forth between Los Angeles and New York City for her regular appearances on NBC's *Today* show, and she was training eight to ten clients a day, starting at 5 A.M. and finishing with her last client by dinnertime.

It was no wonder that she was at her physical peak. Kathy is 5 feet, 8 inches tall. At that time she weighed about 145 pounds and her body had only 11 percent body fat. That's less than half the average woman's body fat content. Kathy had great endurance, great strength, and a great shape.

After we chatted for a few minutes, Kathy announced to me that she was pregnant—with twins! Of course, I was thrilled for her and for Billy. But I had to admit I was curious, too. How was this fabulous body going to be transformed?

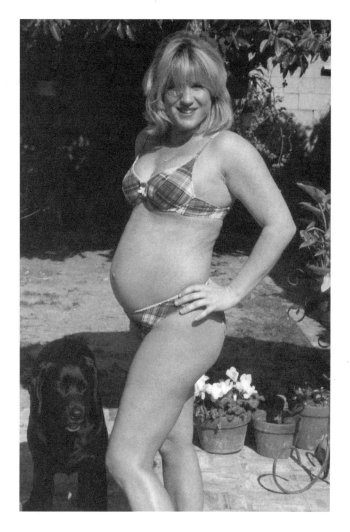

It was a question that had surprising answers. As time went by, Kathy's weight increased steadily. At 12 weeks, she weighed 158 pounds. At 24 weeks, she weighed 191 pounds. When she was 36 weeks pregnant, she weighed 215 pounds. Her body was swollen—even her tongue was enlarged—and all her muscle definition from the hips up had disappeared. When she walked into the hospital to give birth, she weighed 218 pounds. That's a total gain of 73 pounds!

Because she was carrying twins, Kathy's pregnancy had presented a bigger physical challenge than if she were carrying one baby. Her weight gain, while significant, was not unhealthy for a woman who was carrying twins. The extra weight was certainly a burden for someone who was used to a highly physically active daily routine, and because of all that extra weight, not only did she have trouble exercising but even something as simple as breathing became difficult. Adding this to the fact that twins present a higher risk of complications (such as premature delivery and smaller birth weights), Kathy had to be extremely cautious about any and all of her physical activities.

She curtailed her physical activity drastically. Instead of working out with all her clients, she found ways to limit her participation in their workouts. She started handing them their weights rather than lifting the weights along with them. She would demonstrate an exercise but stop short of actually doing it. She reduced her client load and she rested whenever possible. Basically, she listened to whatever her body told her and she acted accordingly.

By the time Kathy became pregnant, she had already listened to what many of her pregnant and postpregnant clients had told her about their bodies. She had personally trained quite a few of them, including some of her celebrity clients, throughout their pregnancies and postpregnancies. And, as a seasoned professional, she modified familiar moves and created new routines that best accommodated the needs of her pregnant and postpregnant clients.

With the help of what she learned from Michelle Pfeiffer, Jami Gertz, Sheryl Berkoff Lowe, Harriet Posner, and Rita Wilson Hanks, as well as from her own experiences, Kathy Kaehler designed the workouts that became *Primetime Pregnancy*.

Because we believe in the importance of physical fitness at all stages of our lives, we urge you to make cardiovascular exercise and muscle toning a lifetime habit. You don't have to be a Hollywood star to recognize the impact that feeling good and looking good has

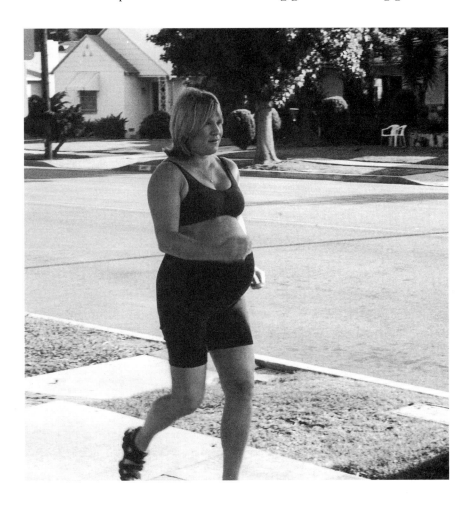

on your life. But you do have to work at it. Everybody does.

We know it takes more than our urging to get you on your feet and working out consistently, but we thought we'd share with you some motivating thoughts that Kathy's clients shared with us.

In *Primetime Bodies*, we told you how far Michelle Pfeiffer will go to keep fit. Even when she's shooting a picture, she gets up at 4:30 in the morning to get in a full workout with Kathy before she goes off to work, where she puts in 12 hours a day on a movie set, and then comes home and gets busy being a wife and mother before preparing for her next day's work.

Michelle works hard at working out because she *wants* to. When she was pregnant with her son, John, she could have easily used her pregnancy as an excuse to cut back on her training or even stop it altogether. She could, in fact, at any time revert to her old way of working out more or less when she feels like it, as opposed to regimenting herself, like we're asking you to do. But Michelle is in a place where we'd like you to go. She's got the right attitude.

Here's where she got it. When she took the role of Catwoman in *Batman Returns*, she was facing a four-month shooting schedule that had her wearing a skintight, highly

revealing cat suit costume. Never disciplined before about her workouts, she came to the realization that she had better change her workout habits. So she started working with Kathy for at least an hour every day. It wasn't particularly easy to get into that habit, but once she did, Michelle said working out daily made her feel and look so much better that each day motivated her to do another day. Quickly, her new habit took hold.

Now, she says, no matter how painful it is to get up early to work out, she pushes herself to do it because without it she does not have the same energy level and she looks more tired when she doesn't work out. Michelle believes, "Whatever I lose from that extra hour's sleep, I gain in energy throughout the day."

Michelle Pfeiffer has now been doing this disciplined workout schedule for over five years and she thinks her longevity is the key to longevity. "Once you feel the effects of looking and feeling better for that long, you want to keep feeling the effects. You don't want to stop. You can't stop."

Sheryl Berkoff Lowe, who is married to actor Rob Lowe, said that, when she was pregnant and working out with Kathy, the regular exercise lifted her spirits.

"As a pregnant woman, you feel heavy on your feet and you feel like you've got a weight strapped on you. You have to be in the psychology of working out because when you're pregnant you don't see results and changes so fast. But when I did [work out] I felt emotionally thinner. I felt like I was doing something for my body and mind by releasing toxins."

After each of her two sons was born, Sheryl admitted that working out "was a bitch. You have to push yourself really hard. You're up at night and you're breast-feeding and you're tired. But I do have an ego so I feel like I have to make it work. I know that working out not only got me back into shape after each baby was born but it also made me feel calmer and more centered."

Harriet Posner, a high-powered entertainment litigator, says exercise is the best stress reliever she knows. Intense exercise, for her, is a form of meditation, and when she experiences it, it helps her tremendously in her work. As for getting back into shape after her pregnancy, Harriet is convinced about the positive correlation between exercise and recovery. "There is no question, after the baby came, working out helped me recover faster and it gave me

an outlet for the emotional and physical changes I was undergoing."

Rita Wilson Hanks found that working out during her pregnancy and after her babies were born gave her a big boost. Her lower-body strength helped ease her deliveries, and while she has a natural propensity toward being thin, she doesn't have a natural propensity toward strong muscles. She really has to work at it. For instance, she worked diligently on strengthening her upper body. All those overhead presses and reverse flys worked wonders at keeping her from aching and feeling exhausted from lifting and holding her baby.

Rita also knows the importance of routine in a successful workout program. Even when she's on the road or on location, or tired from her demanding days as a wife and mother, she finds a way to work in her exercises because exercise for her is an hour of fun, especially when she adds variety to her workouts.

In *Primetime Pregnancy*, we want to help motivate you to get into the habit and feel the effects of regular workouts and to have fun while you're doing them. We know that if you're in good shape while you're pregnant you have a better chance of getting back into

Mom's Muscles

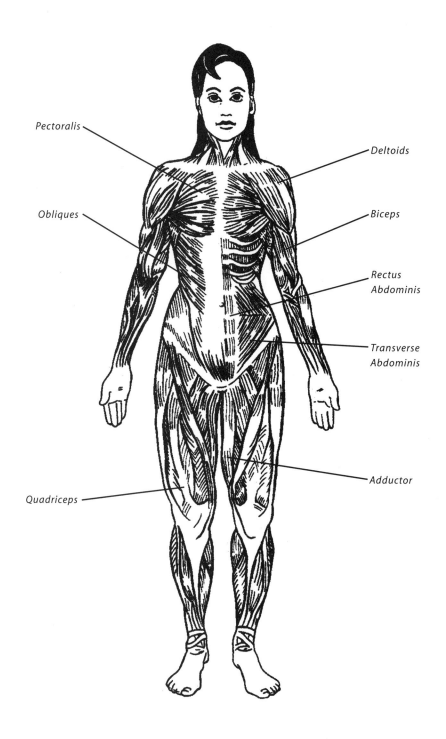

Pectoralis

Deltoids

Obliques

Biceps

Rectus
Abdominis

Transverse
Abdominis

Adductor

Quadriceps

Mom's Muscles

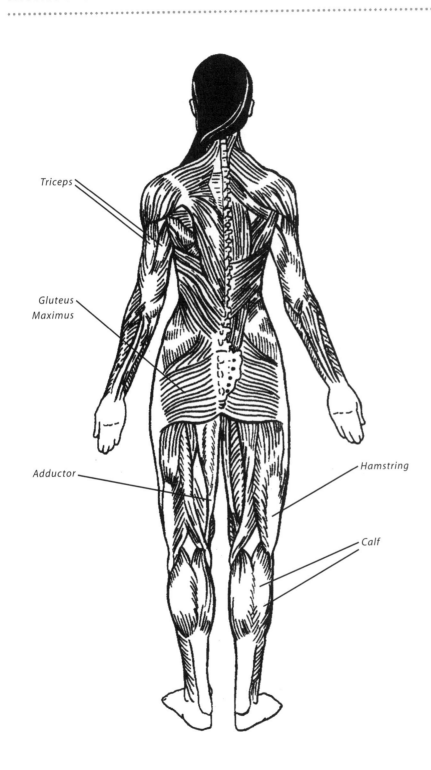

Triceps

Gluteus
Maximus

Adductor

Hamstring

Calf

great shape after you deliver. We think the hardest part of working out is working out. So with this in mind, we've created exercises and exercise combinations that are designed for maximum effect. As usual, the routines are designed for variety. We know the limitations on your time, so they're grouped for convenience—wherever possible we have all the floor work together and all the weights work together.

Also, we urge you to divide your workout throughout the day or night. That way, even if you don't have a single large block of time for yourself, you can accomplish short periods of exercise rather than avoiding exercise altogether.

We use props in our workouts and each workout in this book is preceded by a list of the props you will need for that day's or month's work. They include a straight-back chair, hand weights, and a rubber exercise band, which you can buy in any sporting-goods store. If you prefer, you can use an old pair of panty hose or tights instead of the exercise band. Basically, you need material that is flexible. It should provide you with firm resistance as it expands from its unstretched to its fully stretched state. We think you should do our workout programs in front of a mirror. Not only are

you your best audience but you're your best critic. You should constantly evaluate your positioning. To be effective, you need proper form.

We think music acts as a catalyst in working out. Much like the score in a movie, music can move the action forward. We suggest you try any of Madonna's songs. Melissa Etheridge and Sheryl Crow are also good choices. If you have a favorite artist that makes you feel good, by all means use his or her music as background for your workout.

As in *Primetime Bodies*, we draw parallels between acting and working out. We do that because there *are* parallels: you need a good script to follow, you need to work hard at giving an effective performance, and the results bring kudos.

And, actors learn to tap into their instincts and use those instincts when they act. You, too, should be listening to your instincts when it comes to how you treat your body throughout your pregnancy. Do whatever you can do comfortably. Push yourself to achieve the goals we've set only if you can do them without excessive strain and certainly without peril to you or your baby. And remember: consult your physician before you start any workout program.

Everyone works at her own pace and according to her own ability. We have given you a program that is challenging, even downright difficult at times. For example, there are times (at least five months after the baby is born) when we ask you to do as many as 150 repetitions (reps) of various abdominal exercises. Not everyone will be able to do 150 reps. Michelle still doesn't do 150 abs moves in a workout. She does 50. Rita, who hates abs work, does 200 reps of various exercises while Jami Gertz finds 400 reps are more within her range. It's not the number of abs exercises or the number of repetitions you do of any exercise. It's how effectively and diligently you do them.

Oh, by the way, on some days Kathy doesn't do any crunches while on other days, when she's working with a lot of clients, she does from 800 to 900 crunches in a 12-hour period.

If you're looking for another word of encouragement, we'd like to give it to you before you move on to your workouts.

Sheryl Lowe, before she became a full-time mother, was a full-time makeup artist working in the entertainment field. She worked with Michelle on *Frankie and Johnnie*, which was before Michelle shot *Batman Returns*. As does everyone, Sheryl thought Michelle quite beautiful. And she thought Michelle was certainly in good shape. "Then when I saw her in *Batman*, I said, 'I want what she does!'"

Sheryl got what she wanted when she started working out with Kathy. Now, you can have what Michelle, Sheryl, Rita, Jami, and Harriet all do. You can have Kathy right here in *Primetime Pregnancy*. And that should, could, and will make you look and feel the best that you can be.

Once you achieve that state of mind and being, you will feel like a star. Good luck!

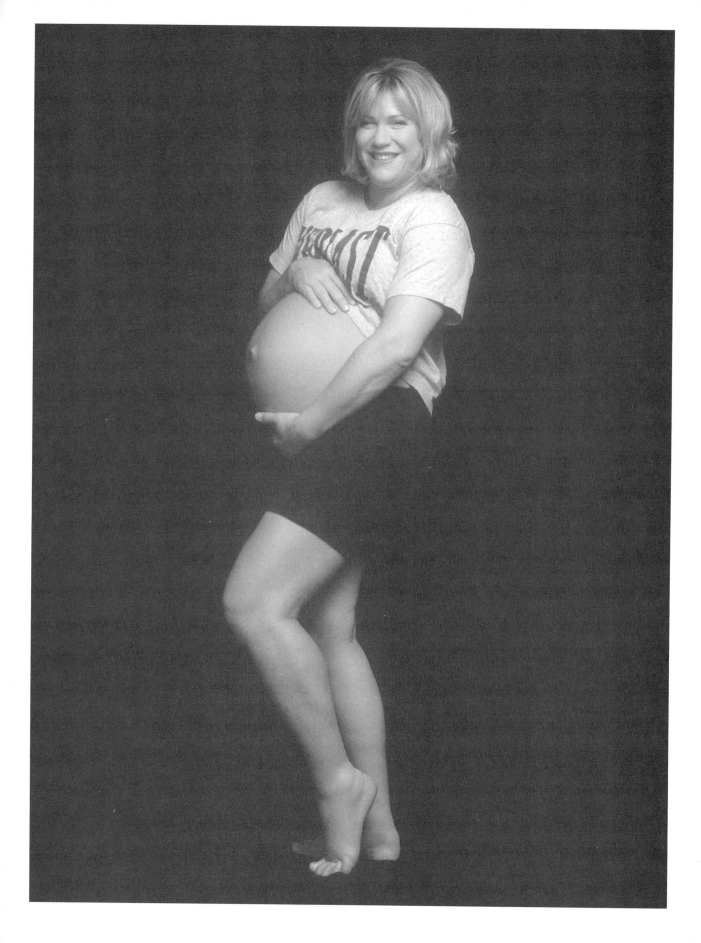

Primetime Pregnancy

One

Signs of Life

Pregnancy—Your First Months

There's no doubt about it . . . pregnancy is the prime time of your life. No matter who you are or what you do for 280 days, wherever you go, you will be center stage. The excitement and anticipation of bringing a new life into the world is contagious. Even strangers are likely to have a reaction to your new status. Until now, your body belonged only to you. Now, not only does it belong to the new life that is growing inside you, but your appearance invites the interest and curiosity of friends, family, and strangers alike.

For the first few months, however, there is little clue to the outer world as to what is happening in your inner world. You, of course, are keenly aware of the changes going on in your body, which is now on hormonal turbo charge.

From the very first weeks of your pregnancy, your body is producing lots of hormones that are needed to grow and nurture your baby. Those hormones have their physical and emotional effects on you. Your breasts begin to get bigger and somewhat sore. You may crave certain foods or develop a distaste for foods that you normally like. You may have "morning sickness" any time of day and feel tired.

By the ninth through twelfth weeks, your weight could start creeping up, even though your appetite may have been tempered by feelings of nausea from morning sickness. You might be urinating more frequently, you could have a little swelling in your feet and ankles, and you're still feeling tired.

These are general changes and not everyone feels them. Kathy felt great for the first few months of her pregnancy. She had no morning sickness and never felt tired. She kept her full load of clients, working out six to eight hours a day, doing everything with them from walking on the treadmill with Michelle Pfeiffer early in the morning to doing step aerobics with Julianne Phillips midday to riding the bike with Lisa Kudrow in the evening.

Jami Gertz did not do as well as Kathy in the early stage of either of her two pregnancies. She was so terribly nauseated in her first trimester that she would walk into the gym to meet Kathy, but before she could even start a warm-up, she'd excuse herself and go throw up. Then, even though she didn't feel great, she'd do her full hour workout with Kathy, albeit at a slower pace. Her morning sickness and tiredness lasted until her fourth month when, like a lot of women, she

began to feel more energized and could put a little more vigor into her workout.

Sheryl Lowe was working as a makeup artist on a film throughout the first three months of her first pregnancy. She was putting in her typically long days of production, but 15 hours a day on her feet was made exceptionally taxing by her ever present and severe morning sickness. She credits working out with helping her get past the discomfort because it took her mind off the nausea.

Harriet Posner's demanding work as a high-powered litigator in the field of entertainment law requires a great deal of energy and stamina. Always physically active—she was on her college tennis team—Harriet started working out with Kathy two months before she became pregnant with her second child. Kathy kept Harriet on a cardio training and weight-lifting program even though Harriet felt constantly enveloped by a blanket of tiredness throughout her first trimester. Listening to her body, Harriet didn't push quite as hard as she was accustomed to, but she didn't give up even one workout session with Kathy.

The same was true for Michelle Pfeiffer. Prior to becoming pregnant she was running four to five miles a day, two days a week. Soon after she became pregnant, she eased up on the running. She still worked out five days a week, but she cut back on the running to three miles a day once or twice a week. She did step aerobics, rode the recumbent bike, or walked on the treadmill the rest of the week. When she was four months pregnant, she stopped running altogether and started walking. As Michelle's pregnancy progressed, Kathy would make adjustments in Michelle's workout to fit her body's signals.

Each of these high-profile Hollywood women had several things in common. Each was physically fit before she became pregnant, and each woman paid close attention to what her body was telling her once she was pregnant and modified her workout accordingly. Each woman knew her life was being changed by her pregnancy and each was determined to maintain as much control as possible over her relationship with her body and fitness. All of these women—with the exception of Kathy—maintained an exercise program throughout their entire pregnancies. None of these women were using exercise to lose weight and none of them went against their doctor's advice. They

all worked out because it made them feel better. Regular exercise heightened their morale, made them feel stronger and more in control, and, as their pregnancies progressed, made them less vulnerable to some of the aches and pains many pregnant women get—like backaches, shoulder and neck strain, and leg and abdominal cramps.

For a lot of women, regular exercise also helps reduce bloating and swelling associated with pregnancy. Michelle is certainly one of those women. At the end of the shooting schedule of her movie *Dangerous Minds*, she was nearly seven months pregnant, and we challenge anyone to watch the movie and see if you are able to detect the fact that she was pregnant at all. Yet, Michelle gained a total of 28 pounds during her pregnancy.

The goal of exercise during pregnancy is to sustain a safe level of fitness. There are by-products to pregnancy fitness: it makes you feel good, and it makes you look good throughout your pregnancy (hopefully as good as Michelle!). Based on our own experience, as well as from information gathered by medical experts, women who are physically fit have more energy and better stamina during labor. Also, physically fit moms-to-be generally have a much easier time getting back into shape after their babies are born.

As much as you want exercise to help make you look good and feel good, you have to *act* good when it comes to pregnancy exercise. Every newly pregnant mom should practice certain precautions as soon as she feels those early signs of life.

If you didn't exercise a lot before pregnancy, you shouldn't take on any strenuous activity for more than 15 to 20 minutes once you become pregnant. If you were active pre-pregnancy, you can exercise longer—up to an hour if your body responds without warning signs (see the list of warning signs on page 33). It's important to avoid jerky, bouncy, or high-impact movements. That's because during pregnancy the hormone relaxin causes your ligaments to relax and your joints to soften and stretch. This makes you more vulnerable to injury, and that vulnerability increases as your pregnancy progresses.

In our pregnancy workouts, we're going to recommend you use light weights in some of our exercises. We suggest you use weights *only* if you have done so in the past. If you've followed our *Primetime Bodies* workouts, weights are a familiar tool for you. Using weights gives you added resistance, and by working with that added resistance, you develop more strength. Throughout your pregnancy, with the added weight of your growing belly and your enlarged breasts, you'll feel some strain on your lower and upper back and on your shoulders. Working with hand weights will help strengthen those areas. And, according to some experts, women who lift weights during pregnancy may have more energy, more restful nights, fewer aches, and more self-confidence. After the baby is born, you'll be glad you lifted those weights. The added strength in your upper body will serve you well when you're picking up and setting the baby down day and night.

We recommend you exercise at least three times a week during your pregnancy. You can exercise as many as six times a week as long as you're feeling fine and you make adjustments according to your body's needs. For instance, as you gain weight your body will respond more quickly (your heart will beat faster) to whatever exercise you're doing; when you feel that effect, you should slow down. A lot of exercise instructors will tell you to stay at your target heart rate when you exercise. We're not as concerned with the number of beats your heart is beating per minute as we are with your perceived exertion rate.

You should be able to carry on a conversation when you exercise at a comfortable pace. If you can string together four words without gulping for air, you're fine. If you gulp air with each word, the intensity of your exercise is too great and you should slow down. If you're on a walk, ask yourself if you can keep up the pace for 20 more minutes. If the answer is yes, you're working at the right intensity. If you think you can only make it another two minutes, you're pushing too hard and you should slow down.

The important thing here is to be active. If you spend nine months as an exercise dropout, remaining sedentary on the sofa or walking only from your front door to your car door, you're bound to lose lean body tissue and gain fat. Of course, that will make it harder for you to get back in shape postpregnancy, but it will also make you feel sluggish during your pregnancy.

Exercise makes you feel like you're a part of the world, a participant in life. It's good for your overall health and attitude. It's why women like Jami and Michelle and Harriet and Sheryl are primetime figures. They know how important it is to keep center stage and not fade into the background. Exercise is good for their self-esteem; it's good for

their future and it will be for yours, too.

As you get further into your pregnancy, you're going to feel more clumsy and less able to make moves as readily or as steadily. Your balance and speed will be directly affected by your size and the shift in your center of gravity. You might have to walk instead of run or use a stationary bike indoors instead of a road bike on the less predictable outdoor terrain. Running or walking on a treadmill will also lessen the chance you might trip on a curb or uneven ground. If you've been taking step classes, you can continue as long as you're comfortable but you should lessen the impact you're used to. So, if you've been using two risers, use one or none—do the step class on the floor. The same goes for aerobics classes. Make sure you do low impact aerobics. It keeps you closer to the ground and there's less impact on your joints.

Be careful about wearing the right shoes. Make sure they give you good support and, if your feet are swollen, don't hesitate to put on a bigger size shoe for comfort. And wear a good supportive bra. Soon after she became pregnant, Kathy started wearing a special support bra 24 hours a day and two months after the twins were born, she was still wearing a good support bra 24 hours a day. The bra helped lessen the strain of the extra weight on her back and shoulders.

Swimming is another aerobic exercise that's good for you while you're pregnant. Swimming uses a lot of your muscles, stretching and toning them, and all the while, the water is supporting your weight.

And speaking of water, be sure to drink plenty of it before you exercise, while you're exercising, and after you're through. This will help keep your body cool, which is healthier for you and your growing baby.

Remember never to exercise on an empty stomach and never to exercise immediately after eating. Your body needs fuel to burn fuel. Have a snack about a half hour to an hour before you work out. The snack can be a slice of whole wheat toast, a banana, an apple, or any high-carbohydrate, low-fat food; these will give you added energy and can even help fight morning sickness.

The exercise routine we have designed for you to do during your pregnancy focuses on the muscle groups that need to be strengthened to help accommodate the changes in your body. We will help you work to keep your body strong during pregnancy, get it into better shape in those key areas that should

help ease your labor, and make it easier for you to get it back in shape after the birth of your baby.

Notes on a Couple of Primetime Positions

There's going to be a lot of talk about your uterus and your pelvic floor throughout your pregnancy. Your growing baby is inside your uterus and your uterus is supported by your pelvic floor. The pubo-coccygeal, or PC, muscle, surrounds the opening of the vagina and covers the entire pelvic floor from the pubic bone to the tailbone. Since your uterus grows to about 1,000 times its normal size, you can understand that your supporting muscles have to perform what is for them a Herculean task. A vaginal delivery will greatly stretch your pelvic floor muscles and could someday lead to incontinence and a prolapsed uterus. These conditions are avoidable if you start working now on strengthening your PC muscle.

About 50 years ago, Dr. Arnold Kegel recognized the importance of fortifying the PC muscle, and he created some exercises to help develop PC muscle strength. Because of their importance throughout your pregnancy, during the birthing process, and postpartum, we have included pelvic–floor strengthening exercises in both our pregnancy and postpregnancy workouts.

You can locate your PC muscle easily. While you're urinating, stop your flow of urine. It's the PC muscle that contracts to do this. Practice this starting and stopping of urine flow so you can get the feeling of this muscle. Try some stronger and weaker contractions until you can contract this muscle when you're not urinating. Once you've got the hang of these, do not do them while you're urinating because you'll run the risk of urinary-tract infections.

Almost every woman in America, it seems, is concerned with the shape of her abs. At this point in your life, you're concerned, too, but for a new set of reasons. With your uterus growing and adding bulk to your abdominal area, your stomach muscles can become strained as they stretch. During pregnancy, many women develop a mild separation of the rectus abdominis muscle. This is the long muscle that runs from your chest to your pubic bone (see the schematic drawing on page xii). When the two halves of this muscle separate, it's called diastasis recti (see page 32). You can keep this separation

at a minimum by strengthening your transverse abdominis muscle. The transverse is the muscle that runs across the abdominals (see the schematic drawing on page xvi). It is attached to your bottom six ribs and to your recti in front. This muscle will help you when you push your baby out in delivery, and it will help you get your abs back into shape after the baby is born.

We will work to strengthen your abs with a breathing exercise we call the "accordion." The accordion will also help relieve lower back pain and help your posture, which will be strongly affected by the weight of your uterus tilting your pelvis forward and away from your spinal column.

Now that we've given you the notes on your pregnancy workout script, let's roll. Action, please.

The Warm-Up

Before you start our strengthening exercises, we suggest you warm up for no less than five minutes with our warm-up routine. If you're feeling up to it, you can do up to a full hour of the aerobic activity or activities of your choice, ranging from walking to running, swimming to step class.

If you choose to do a basic warm-up only, you can try the one

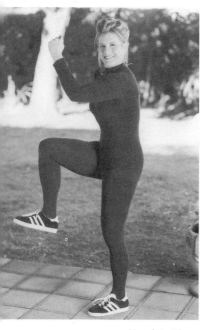

March in Place

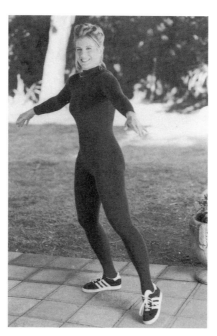

Move Arms and Legs Laterally

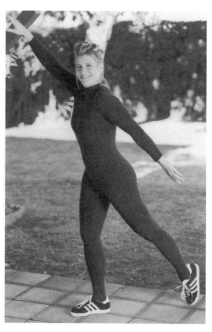

Swing Arms, Extend Legs Back

we first gave you in *Primetime Bodies* or you can follow this simple warm-up, which will get your blood circulating and get your mind into primetime focus.

Start by marching in place. As you alternately lift each foot slightly off the floor, lift the opposite arm up over your head, with your fingertips pointing toward the ceiling (as you lift your right foot, your left arm goes up; as you lift your left foot, your right arm goes up). If you feel comfortable, especially in the earlier stages of your pregnancy, lift your knees as high as your waist. But even if you can lift your feet only slightly off the floor, you will get your blood circulating. The lift and stretch of your arms toward the ceiling will also increase the cardio benefits of this move.

Count each lift of the right and left foot as 1 repetition (rep). Do 10 reps to complete 1 set. Do 3 sets.

Now, again in place, you will do a lateral move with your feet while raising your arms laterally as well. Step your right foot and leg out to your right side as you lift both of your arms out to the side so that they are shoulder level and parallel to the floor. Lower your arms as you bring your feet back together. Now step your left foot and leg out to your left side as you lift your arms, again to shoulder level and parallel to the floor. Lower your arms and bring your feet together before you make your next move to the right. Count the move right and left as 1 rep. Remember to keep your knees soft as you step from side to side. Do 10 of these reps to complete 1 set. Do 3 sets.

The third move in this simple warm-up has you alternating your legs back as you swing your arms forward and back. Try not to tilt forward; keep your torso tall as you start with your right leg, stepping back behind you with just your toe touching the floor. Be careful not to kick your leg back but, rather, make this a controlled move. As you place your right leg back, squeeze your right glut and swing your left arm forward.

Now do the same move with your left leg back and your right arm forward. When you place your left leg behind you, squeeze your left glut. You will feel this move working both your butt and your hamstrings as you get the cardio benefit from swinging your arms and moving your legs.

Count the move with your right and your left legs back as 1 rep. Do 10 of these reps to complete 1 set. Do 3 sets.

The last move in this warm-up is a shoulder roll. Stand with your feet slightly less than shoulder-width apart, with your knees slightly bent and your hands loose at your sides. Lift your shoulders up and move them back and down in a rolling motion. A full roll is 1 rep. Repeat this roll 10 times.

If you feel warmed up after going through each of these four moves, you can go on to your workout. One trip through these moves after a walk outside or on the treadmill should make you feel ready to start your workout. But if you haven't done any other aerobics and you feel that you'd like to get a little warmer before you start working your muscles, go through the entire circuit a second or even a third time.

Remember, your "ready" point is relative to your fitness level and the progression of your pregnancy. If you're really fit, you get warmed up faster. If you're

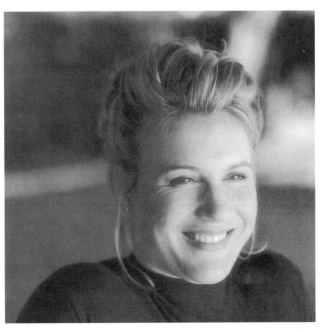

Shoulder Roll

really pregnant, you get warmed up faster (oxygen consumption increases 15 to 20 percent during pregnancy and increased progesterone levels raise your normal breathing rate by 45 percent). Pay attention to what your body is telling you and move accordingly.

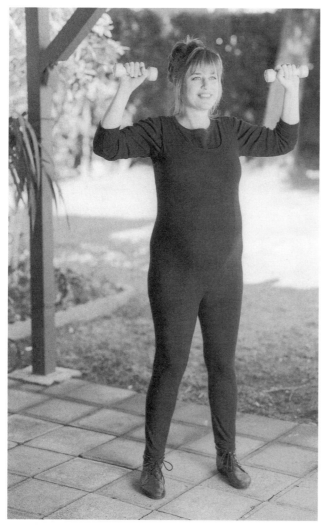

Overhead Press

The Monday Workout

This is the first of your three workouts for the week. The time you devote to this workout is up to you. You can go through the entire circuit once and call it a day. You can go through the full circuit and then repeat it. You can add repetitions to a move that works a body part that you feel needs more strengthening.

As for the weights, we're recommending you go light—3 pounds. If you're used to working with heavier weights, you can try them here. Remember, though, you've got extra weight built in now and your joints are a little looser from the relaxin hormone; you want to be extra careful not to strain yourself because that could lead to injury.

You need a chair for these exercises, so have one handy, and if you're not working out on a carpet, a mat or a thick towel should be close by for you to use in your floor work.

Overhead Press

We'll start in a standing position with the overhead press. You're going to need weights for this exercise. Muscles get stronger when you push them to resist a movement they ordinarily do. With this movement you'll strengthen your shoulders or deltoids by pressing weights up.

Stronger shoulders will help you stand straighter even though the added weight of your breasts pulls you forward.

Stand with your feet shoulder-width apart. Your knees are slightly bent and your pelvis is in a neutral position. Take a weight in each hand and, with the palms of your hands facing forward, start by bending your arms at the elbow. Position your elbows so they are parallel with your shoulders. Raise your arms up overhead as you exhale, pulling in on your abs. Hold your weights up for a beat; then inhale as you return your arms to their original position, which is elbows at shoulder level. You have completed 1 rep. Now repeat the overhead press.

Do 8 reps of this exercise to complete 1 set.

Sit-Down Squat

Sit in your chair but push yourself a little forward so you're not leaning against the back of the chair. You may continue to hold on to your weights or you can place them down on the floor away from your feet, so they'll be handy for the next move.

If you hold on to your weights, hold them loosely in your hands with your arms at your sides,

palms facing in toward you. If you do this exercise without weights, your arms and hands are positioned the same: down at your sides, palms facing in.

Lift yourself off the chair, squeezing your gluts together as you lift. At the same time, lift your arms and extend them forward, so they are parallel to the floor when you're standing. Make sure you press your heels into the

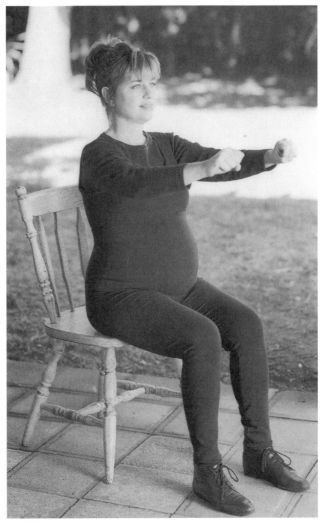

Sit-Down Squat

floor as you stand. Your knees should not bend forward beyond your toes.

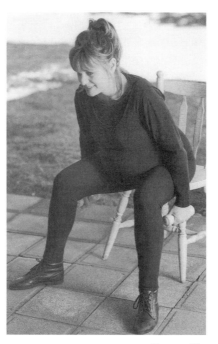

Reverse Fly

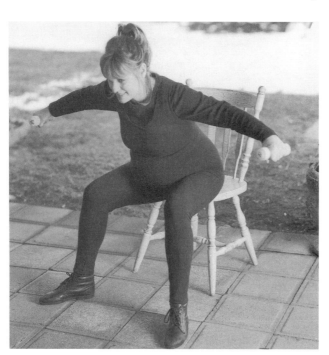

Sit back down in the chair, again making sure your weight is in your heels and your upper body is straight. Do not bend forward from the waist. As you sit back in the chair, lower your arms down again to their starting position at your sides.

This is not as easy as it sounds because of the extra weight you're carrying. But it is a great exercise for strengthening your quads and toning your gluts. We're using the chair, rather than having you do free standing squats, to give you a measure of security in case your balance is a little off because of the shift in your center of gravity.

Count each move up and down as 1 rep. Do 10 reps of these squats.

Reverse Fly

You're going to stick with your chair on this one. The reverse fly works your upper back and rear deltoids. This is an important area to strengthen because you'll be bending over a lot as you feed and hold the baby.

Sit squarely on the seat and pick up your weights. Your feet are planted on the floor in front of you and your knees are bent so that your upper and lower leg form a right angle. Lean forward so that your torso comes down over your quads. You can rest lightly on your quads but do not round your shoulders. Hold your weights loosely in your hands. The palms of your hands are facing in. Your face is looking down.

Keep your back flat as you raise your arms out to your sides. Your elbows are slightly bent as you "fly" your arms back squeezing your shoulder blades together. Make sure your elbows end up level with your upper back. They should go no farther. Now lower your arms back down to your sides and repeat.

Count each lift of the arms up and down as 1 rep. Do 8 reps of these reverse flys.

Side Leg Lift

This exercise is good for toning your outer thigh or your gluteus medius, which is a spot where women tend to put on weight. You have to go down to the floor for this one.

Start by lying on your left side with your left arm extended on the floor in line with your shoulder. Rest your head on your hand. Bend your knees and bring

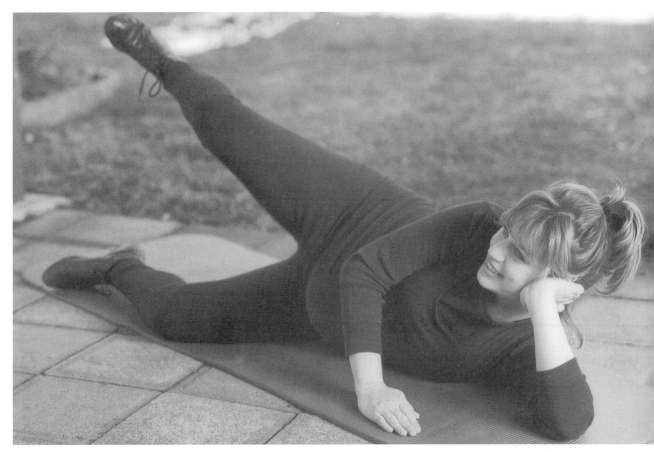

Side Leg Lift

them up toward your chest, stopping when your knees are at an angle to your hips that is halfway between 45 and 90 degrees.

Your hips and legs are stacked so that the inside of your top knee, which is your right knee, looks down on the inside of your left knee. Place your right arm out in front of your chest for support.

Now lift your right leg, exhaling and pulling in your abs as you do. Because you want to isolate the outer thigh, you have to keep steady, taking care not to roll backward or forward. Squeeze your butt as you lower your leg and inhale at the same time. Do not rest your right leg on your left leg. Lift again.

Count each lift and lower as 1 rep. Do 15 reps and switch sides so you can repeat this exercise with your left leg on top.

Now, lying on your right side, your right arm is outstretched in line with your shoulder. Rest your head on your right arm and bring in your legs with knees bent again at an angle to your hips. Lift your left leg up, taking care not to roll backward or forward. Exhale when you lift, pulling in on your abs, and when you lower your leg, squeeze your butt at the same time you inhale.

Do 15 side lifts with your left leg and roll onto your back.

Pelvic Tilt

Lie on your back with your knees bent and your feet flat on the floor. Your heels are about three feet in front of your butt. Your head, neck, and shoulders rest comfortably on the floor while you tilt your pelvis up, squeezing up your lower abs and your butt just off the floor. Do *not* lift your lower back off the floor—just tilt your pelvis up making sure that only your butt is lifting. Squeeze it harder at the top and hold it for a beat, then lower your butt back down onto the floor. Don't rest.

Do 25 reps of the pelvic tilt.

With each tilt, you're strengthening your pelvic floor so it can better withstand the pressure of the increased weight of your uterus and your bladder pushing down. The side benefits of this exercise are that it is good for relieving lower back pain and it helps shape and tone your gluts.

The next exercise works well with the pelvic tilt. In fact, you can do them simultaneously. But for now, let's start with them alone.

Kegel

The pubo-coccygeal (PC) muscle is in the pattern of a figure eight around the openings to the rectum, the vagina, and the urethra. This muscle supports the organs in the pelvis. Those organs are the bowel, the bladder, and the uterus. The PC muscle aids in childbirth, as well as in urination and bowel movements. In each case, to facilitate these movements out of the body, the PC muscle has to release by stretching. It will stretch more easily if it's stronger, so the importance of routinely practicing these kegels—PC strengthening exercises—cannot be too highly stressed.

You can do your PC exercises anytime you want to—while you're waiting in line at the checkout counter in the supermarket, while you're walking down the street, before you get out of bed in the morning, or when you're doing the pelvic tilts. It's up to you.

For now, since you're already on the floor, try doing your kegels while you're in the same position as you were for the pelvic tilt. Your back, neck, and head are resting comfortably. Your knees are up at almost a right angle to your pelvis. Now squeeze—as if you're stopping your urine from flowing. Hold that squeeze for one second and then release.

Do 25 kegels then stand up and get ready to squeeze and release your accordion.

Accordion

You're now breathing for two . . . and your body needs more oxygen to supply you and your growing baby. In *Primetime Bodies*, we told you about the importance that proper breathing plays in an actor's performance. You may not know it but just before she walks on stage or just before the camera rolls, the actor takes control of her character through acute concentration that is coupled with her taking a deep breath. As you prepare for your role in childbirth, it's just as important for you to take control of your breathing because breathing right will make you healthier and stronger.

These accordions will help reduce the risk of developing diastasis recti—that separation of the long stomach muscle—by strengthening your abdominal muscles. (See page 32 before doing any abdominal exercises.) The accordions will also help you breathe better. It's a lesson good for a lifetime. The key is to expand your abs on the inhale and pull them in on the exhale. Ready?

Stand with your knees slightly bent and your pelvis tilted slightly forward. Now pretend that you have an accordion in your belly. It's placed back to front, that is, one handle is against your spine and the other against your abs.

Take a deep breath in through the belly to expand your accordion all the way. Now exhale, pulling in until the accordion is halfway closed. The exercise really kicks in here where the accordion is half open and you exhale further to blow all the air out of it and close it. So the exercise is from halfway to closure and each halfway to closure is 1 rep. As for counting reps, to be most effective, count out loud each time you pull back toward your spine.

The rhythm is inhale, exhale, and then small rhythmic exhales, as you do small contractions between the halfway and the closed position. Count each of these smaller exhales as 1 rep. Do 25 reps. Release.

Play On

If you feel you've done enough of a workout for today, you can move on to the cool-down. If you feel like you're just getting started, then do just that. Start again and repeat the entire circuit of

exercises. If, after you've done the exercises a second time and you feel like your job is done for the day, move on to the cool-down. But for all you hearty mothers-to-be, you can go back and repeat any and all of the exercises in this Monday workout.

- Please remember to drink plenty of water.
- Do not continue if you have any of the warning signs (listed on page 33).
- Always cool down.

The Cool-Down

Arm-Leg Opposition

You're on the floor, on your back, with your legs straight and your arms extended. Bend your knees and drop them to your right side. Take your right arm and place it across your chest so that both your arms rest opposite to your bent knees.

You'll feel the stretch in your trunk. Hold the stretch for at least 10 seconds and preferably for 30 seconds. Then switch sides.

Take your knees over to your left side and drop them down so they're resting on the floor. Your arms go in the opposite direction—to your right side. Hold

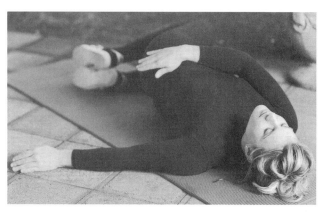

Arm-Leg Opposition

the stretch for 10 to 30 seconds. Release.

Still on your side, use your arms to push yourself up into sitting position.

V-Sit Stretch

Sit up on the floor and open your legs as wide as you can, so they are in a V-shape. Remember, never force a stretch. As you do this stretch more and more often, you'll become more limber and a wider stretch will be easier.

Reach up with your left arm and gently stretch over to your right side and hold. Stretch only as far as you can comfortably go. You can rest your right arm on your thigh. Hold for 10 to 30 seconds. You'll feel this in your pelvis and hamstrings and you'll feel it in your waist.

Release this stretch and repeat it on your other side. Reach up with your right arm and over to your left side. Hold for 10 to 30 seconds and release.

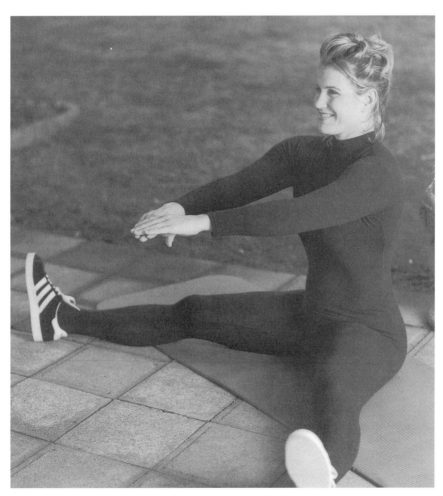

V-Sit Stretch

Complete this stretching exercise by sitting up straight, legs still in the V position. Now, leaning forward so that your torso comes down between your legs, walk your arms forward, stretching from your pelvis. Go only as far forward as you feel comfortable doing. Hold this stretch for 10 to 30 seconds.

Butterfly Stretch

Sit up and bring your feet in toward your body by bending your knees. The soles of your feet should be facing each other and your upper body is straight. You're stretching your inner thighs with this move. Hold the stretch for 10 to 30 seconds and release.

Cat Stretch

Now move on to your hands and knees. Take your back and round up by pulling your abs in toward your spine. Exhale as you pull up on your abs and inhale as you release. Do 6 to 8 reps.

Keeping your arms stretched in front of you, push yourself back into a squatting position with your knees bent. Lower your butt down onto your heels. Hold—again for 10 to 30 seconds. You'll feel the stretch in your shoulders, upper back, and lower back.

Walk your arms back and position your feet flat on the floor so that now you are squatting with your arms hanging at your sides. Hold this for as long as you can, feeling the stretch in your butt, quads, and inner thighs.

Push up to a half standing position by placing one hand on each quad and pushing. Your butt will stick out behind you; your head is looking straight out. Your hands remain on your quads. Now round your back and bring your chin in toward your chest. Release your back into a flat position. Round and release 6 to 8 times.

Butterfly Stretch

Come up to a full standing position and take a deep breath. As you inhale, bring your arms up overhead and when you exhale bring your arms down to your sides.

You're done! Today's performance is over. You can do an encore tomorrow if you wish or wait until Wednesday and follow a new script.

The Wednesday Workout

Once again, you must be sure to warm up before you start your workout. Actors routinely use different techniques— "exercises"—to help them get into character. Most of these acting exercises help the actors to create an emotional environment for their characters to inhabit. You can look at the warm-up as your time to get into character. These few minutes will help you take your mind off everything but you. Right now, you is two, with twice the motivation for staying healthy and fit.

If you're feeling up to it, it's a good idea to stick to a cardio-vascular workout, which would include walking, biking, "stepping," stair climbing, or

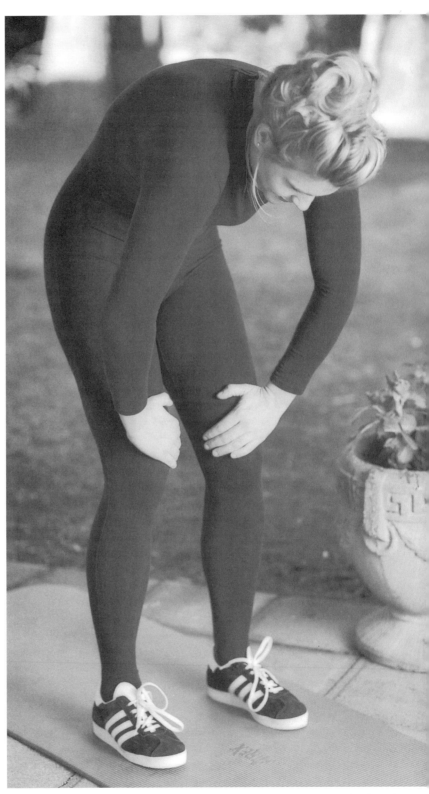

Cat Stretch

swimming. Do one of these activities for five minutes to sixty minutes depending on how fit you are and how you feel on any given day.

If you're up for a five- to ten-minute warm-up, follow our warm-up from Monday. It's on page 7.

When you've completed that warm-up, step into the spotlight. It's showtime!

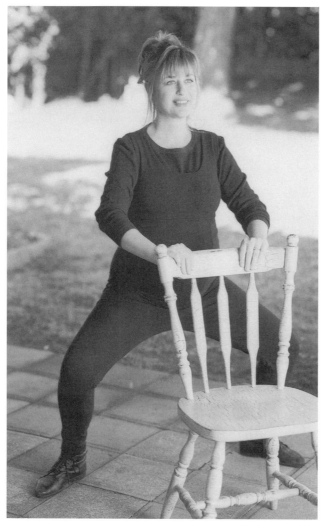

Plié Squat

- Straight-back chair
- Hand weights

Plié Squat

Your first move is going to work your quads and your gluts. You'll use your own body weight for resistance.

Stand with your feet about shoulder-width apart. If you were standing on the face of an imaginary clock, your feet would be at ten o'clock and two o'clock. Your toes are pointed out. Your hands are resting lightly on the back of the chair for balance only.

Lower your body as you bend your knees. Your knees will bend out over your toes until they're in line with your toes. Never let them go any farther. You should be able to see your toes.

Bring your butt down so it's just above your knees. Never let your gluts go lower than your knees because it puts too much strain on your knees.

Keep your weight resting on your heels. Now lift, squeezing your gluts as you come up.

Count each move down and up as 1 rep. Do 10 reps.

Pick up your hand weights.

Military Press

If you're feeling strong enough, you can stand up for this exercise. If you're having any difficulties with balance or you're just more comfortable sitting on a chair, have a seat. Either sitting or standing, this is an upper-body move that works the anterior deltoids (front of your shoulders).

This exercise is similar in its basic movement to the overhead press we did on Monday (see page 10). The difference is the overhead press has your weights meeting directly overhead, which works the middle deltoid. The military press is more forward than overhead.

The basic standing position has your legs shoulder-width apart and your knees slightly bent. With your 3-pound weights—one in each hand, palms facing forward—bend your arms so your hands are level with your shoulders. Now raise your arms up and slightly forward of your head. Your hands and weights meet overhead, in front of your head. Now lower the weights back down to shoulder level.

Count each press up as 1 rep. You don't count the return move. Do 8 of these military presses.

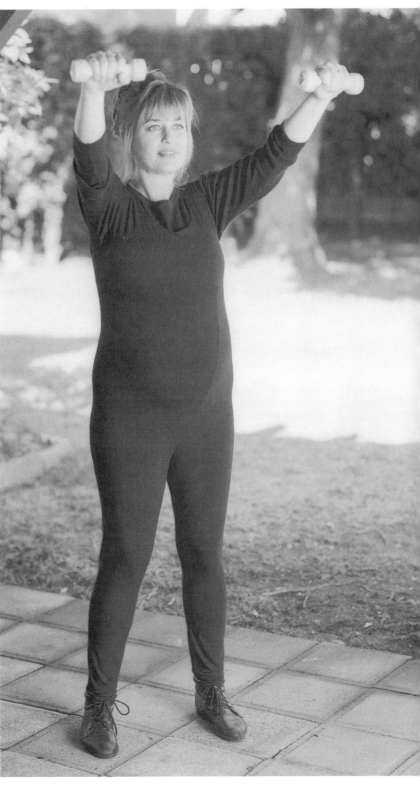

Military Press

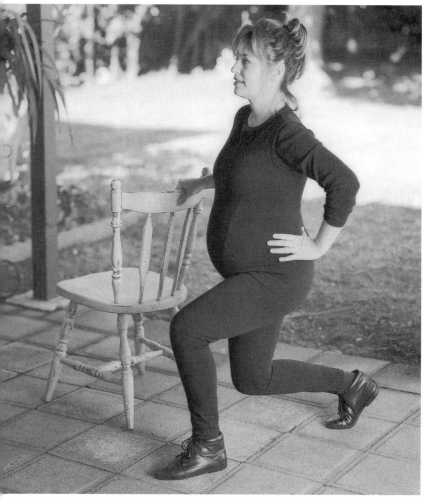

Split Lunge

Make sure your knee is over your ankle—no farther forward than that. Keep the weight on the heel of your front (left) foot. The heel of your back foot is raised off the floor. Press up to the starting position with your left foot still in front of you and your right foot still behind. Bend your knees and lower again.

Do this move for 10 reps.

Switch working legs. Still holding on to the chair with your right hand, step your right foot forward one step and step your left foot back one step. Bend both knees and lower. Keep the weight on the heel of your right leg. Now push back off that heel and return to the starting position.

Do 10 lunges with your right leg forward.

Lateral Raise

Pick up your weights again. Move away from the chair and stand with your legs slightly more than shoulder-width apart, with your knees slightly bent. One weight in each hand, your palms start down at your sides, facing in toward your body. Keeping your elbows slightly bent, simultaneously raise both arms out to your sides, squeezing your shoulder blades together. Do not lift your arms any higher than shoulder level and be careful not to lift your shoulders up to your ears. Lower your arms

Split Lunge

You definitely need the chair for this so you can balance. Stand with your right side next to the back of the chair. Your body forms a "T" with the chair. Rest your right hand lightly on the top of the back of the chair. Now step your left foot forward one step and step your right foot back one step. You are still in a "T" with the chair. Bend both knees and lower.

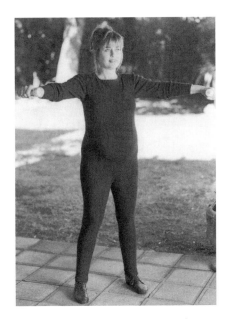

Lateral Raise

back down to your sides. You'll feel this exercise in your shoulders where you're trying to build more strength, which will help you with holding and feeding the baby.

Count each lift up and out to the side as 1 rep. Do 8 reps.

Shoulder Press

Set your weights aside. Stand in the basic position of legs slightly more than shoulder-width apart, knees slightly bent. Lift your shoulders up toward your ears, then back down halfway. Complete the move by pressing your shoulders back down to starting position. The emphasis here is on the *downward press* because this will help you release the tension in your shoulders.

Each shoulder press is done in three counts, making 1 rep. Do 10 reps of each three-count shoulder press.

Pelvic Tilt with Bridge

On Monday, we did pelvic tilts (see page 14). We're going to do them again today but we've made them a little harder by adding a bridge. A bridge is an extra lift of the butt and it gets the lower back into the act by lifting it off the floor.

Lie down on the floor with your head and shoulder blades planted. Bend your knees and bring your feet in until your heels are about three feet from your butt. Now squeeze your gluts and pull in on your lower abs as you lift your gluts off the floor. Add the bridge by lifting your gluts

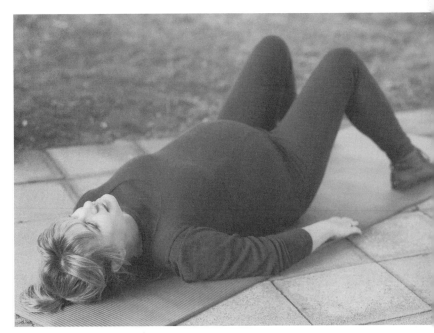

Pelvic Tilt with Bridge

higher, squeezing harder, and lifting your lower back off the floor. Hold at the top for a beat and lower to your starting position.

Count each tilt and bridge as 1 rep. Do 25 reps.

Kegel

We did them on our backs on Monday (see page 14). Now we're going to switch to our sides. Gently come over to your right side, extending your right arm so you can rest your head on that arm. Bend your knees and bring them up slightly, finding a position that's comfortable.

Now, as if you're stopping a flow of urine, squeeze the PC muscle. Hold for 1 second and release. Squeeze again. Do 25 of these kegels and with your left

arm gently push yourself onto your back.

Abdominal Curl

These curls will help strengthen your abs and help keep those long stomach muscles from separating. You're only going to be on your back for about a minute, so you can do this exercise up to your second trimester without difficulty.

On your back, place your hands behind your head and rest your head gently in your hands. Bend your knees and with your feet flat on the floor, bring your feet in toward your butt. Your legs should be in an inverted "V" position.

With your lower back resting on the floor, lift your head and

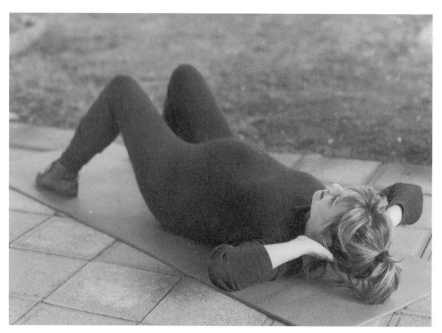

Abdominal Curl

shoulders up and slightly off the floor. Do not pull on your head or neck. You exhale as you lift and your abs contract toward your spine. Now lower your head and shoulders back onto the floor as you inhale. Then lift again.

Count each lift and lower as 1 rep. Do 25 reps.

Accordion

Stand with your knees slightly bent and your pelvis tilted slightly forward. The accordion in your belly is perpendicular to your spine. Take a deep breath into your belly to expand your accordion all the way.

Now exhale, pulling in until the accordion is halfway closed. The exercise starts here: When the accordion is half open, exhale further to blow all the air out of it and close it. Each movement from halfway closed to closed is 1 rep. Count out loud each time you pull back toward your spine.

The rhythm is inhale, exhale, and then a series of 25 rhythmic exhales, which are accompanied by small contractions of the abs.

Today's performance is almost over. If you feel like you haven't given it your all, go back and repeat the entire circuit or repeat just those exercises that you feel target the spot you'd most like to work. Or, if you'd like a change of pace, after you've completed today's workout, go back to Monday's workout and run through that script. Then when you're done, before the curtain comes down for the day, turn to page 16 for the cool-down. Remember, it's important to bring your breathing and heart rate back down to normal. Your heart has been pumping extra blood to your working muscles. The cool-down will keep that blood from pooling in your extremities.

You can do today's routine again tomorrow or take a day off and get ready to meet Friday's challenge.

The Friday Workout

If you're finding you could use yet more challenge in your workout, we suggest that you increase the number of repetitions, or counts, that you do on each move. So, for instance, if an exercise calls for 25 reps, do 30 instead. It would be particularly helpful to you if you could increase your kegels and your accordions. Your PC muscle and your abs are so very important to your delivery and your postpartum shape-up that the more you can do, the better.

We've been calling for 3-pound weights for our upper-body

work. If you feel that you can handle 4- or 5-pound weights, please do. Or, you can alternate between 3, 4, or 5 pounds. In other words, improvise. You do not always have to stick to our script. All we ask is that, if you make changes, please do them carefully and pay attention to what your body is telling you.

We hope you've been able to find time to do some aerobics before you start your workout. Even if you do your walking or biking first, please start our program each day with our warm-up. We have designed this warm-up to maximize the efficiency of the workout that follows.

If you're ready to start, turn to page 7 for our warm-up. If you're using our warm-up alone without any aerobics, you may want to complete the entire warm-up and then repeat it. This will give your body an extra opportunity to get warm and your mind a few extra minutes to shut out the world so you can focus on you.

PROPS

- Straight-back chair
- Hand weights
- Rubber exercise band or panty hose

Plié Leg Lift

Stand facing the back of your chair with your hands resting lightly on the chair. Your legs are slightly more than shoulder-width apart. If you were standing on the face of a clock your feet would be at ten o'clock and two o'clock. Your toes are pointed out.

Keeping your weight in your heels, lower your body, bending your knees so that your torso comes down toward the floor. Your knees come out over your toes as you lower, but make sure you can see your toes. If you can't, you've either bent too far down or your feet are not far enough apart. Your pelvis remains neutral. Do not go down so that your butt is any lower than your knees.

Now lift up and as you do, squeeze your gluts. When your legs are almost straight, stop the lift but keep your knees slightly soft. Keep your right leg in place while you lift your left leg up off the floor. Your foot is flexed as you bend your left knee, lifting it waist high. Lower your leg. This is 1 rep.

Repeat the action by lowering into a plié and pushing up into a leg lift. Do 10 reps. Switch legs.

Again stand behind the back of the chair, both feet on the floor in the ten and two o'clock positions. Lower your torso by bending your knees, then come up, squeezing your gluts as you do. Before you've straightened your left leg, bend your right knee and lift up your right leg so that your knee comes waist high. Lower it. Now lower your body back into the plié position. Each plié and leg lift is 1 rep. Do 10 reps with your right leg.

You will feel these in your inner thighs, your quads, and your gluts.

Triceps Dip

Come around to the front of your chair and stand with your back toward the seat of your chair. Place your hands behind you on the chair seat, keep your arms straight and bring your knees out in front of you, forming right angles with your legs and upper body.

Your fingers face forward and you bend your elbows slightly to where your butt and thighs are level with the chair seat. Dip down so that your butt and your back skim the chair as you lower. Be sure your elbows are pointed back. Go only as far down as is comfortable. Even if you could, do

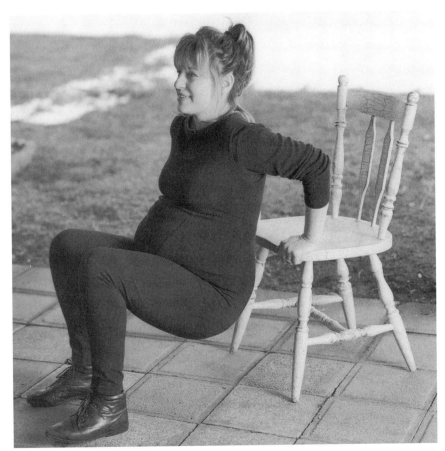

Triceps Dip

not let your butt touch the floor.

Make sure to contract your abs by exhaling as you lift. Each dip and lift is 1 rep. Do 10 reps.

Standing Side Leg Lift

Come back behind the chair and rest your hands lightly on the back of the chair. Place your feet just a couple of inches apart, with your toes facing forward. Bend your knees slightly. Tilt your pelvis a little forward and lift your right leg

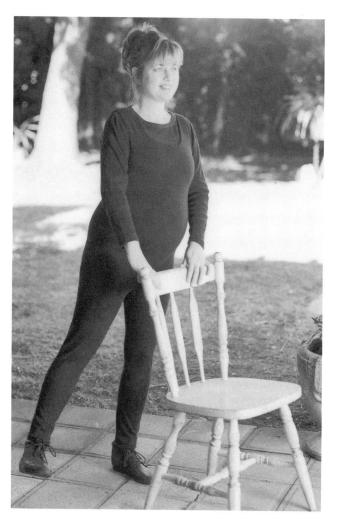

Standing Side Leg Lift

out to the side, flexing your right foot and keeping your toes pointed forward. Squeeze your gluts as you lift. You will not be able to make this a big move since you'll be working against your tilted pelvis. Your flexed foot will come just an inch or two off the floor, then lower your foot back into the starting position. Count each lift to the side and down as 1 rep. Do 15 reps with your right leg lifting, then switch.

Starting with both feet on the floor, a couple of inches apart, check that your pelvis is still tilted forward. Your toes are still pointed forward as you lift your left leg up, getting your foot just off the floor. Your right knee remains slightly bent. Lower your left leg. Do 15 reps.

Biceps Curl

Pick up your weights. Your biceps are most likely the strongest muscles in your arms so you can use heavier weights for this exercise.

Get into the basic position of legs slightly more than shoulder-width apart and your knees slightly bent. With the weights in your hands, start with your palms facing forward. Your hands are down at your sides. As you curl your arms up toward your shoulders, your fists will face your shoulders at the top. Squeeze your

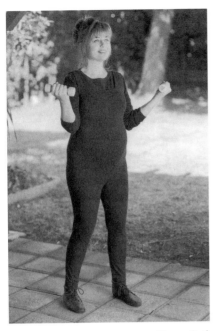

Biceps Curl

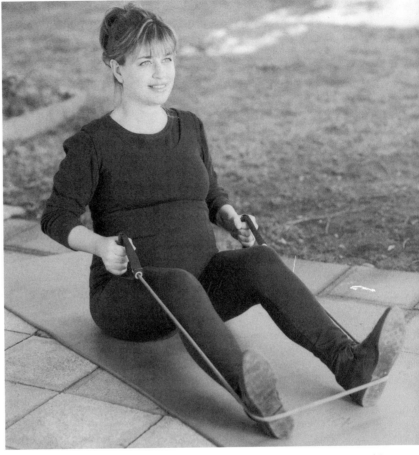

Seated Row

biceps as you curl up and squeeze them as you lower your arms to the starting position.

Count each curl and lower as 1 rep. Do 10 reps.

Seated Row

You're going to need your stretch band or panty hose to create resistance in this move. Sit down on the floor and extend your legs in front of you but do not straighten them. Keep your knees slightly bent. Hold the ends of the band in your hands (if you're using an old pair of panty hose, be sure to hold the waistband in one hand and the two feet of the hose together in the other hand) and run the band or hose under your feet. You will feel the tension in the band created by this stretching. Your palms are facing inward.

Make sure the band is secure in both of your hands as you pull back on it, while keeping your palms facing in and letting your elbows bend back. Pull as far back as you can, feeling the work in your biceps and rear deltoids. Release your arms into their original straight position.

Count each pull back as 1 rep. Do 15 reps.

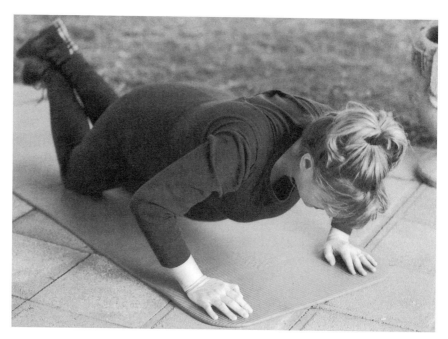

Push-Up

Push-Up

There is nothing like the old-fashioned push-up to best work your arms, chest, and shoulders. So let's take to the floor. Get on all fours, with bent knees and arms extended in a straight line down from your shoulders. Cross your ankles and raise your feet. Your head is forward with your face looking down toward the floor.

Inhale as you lower your body. Keep your back straight and come down as far as you can without touching the floor. As you push back off the floor, exhale and pull in your abs. Squeeze your gluts and make sure your back is straight, not sagging, which is what most people have a tendency to do.

Count each move down as 1 rep. Do 10 reps.

Kegel

Lie down on the floor on your right side. Extend your right arm out and place your head down on your arm. Stack your legs, one on top of the other, and bend your knees slightly. If you're more comfortable, you can place a pillow between your knees. Now, with that same tightening sensation that effects the stop of your urine flow, contract your PC muscle and hold the contraction for 1 second. Release and repeat. Do 25 (or more) kegels.

Pelvic Tilt with Bridge

Gently push yourself onto your back. It's OK—you'll only be there for about a minute. Bend your knees and bring your heels in until they're about three feet from your butt. Contract your abs and squeeze your butt as you tilt your pelvis up and lift your butt off the floor. Hold a beat and release.

Count each tilt as 1 rep. Do 25 reps.

Accordion

We're going to work some more on those abdominal muscles. Pull out the accordion by inhaling a big belly breath and squeeze in on the accordion by blowing out some of the air. About halfway between its full extension and a complete collapse, stop and start a succession of small contractions as you exhale. Count each contraction as 1 rep. Do 25 reps.

If you feel you're ready for more, go back and do the circuit again or do Wednesday's workout or, if you feel creative today, take some moves from each and put them together.

If you've had enough for today, it's time to cool down. Go to page 16 for our cool-down.

Our cool-down is a series of stretches. Stretching lengthens your muscles and increases your flexibility. Even though the progesterone and relaxin in your body are making your joints looser, which could lead to certain injuries, you shouldn't avoid stretching. Just be careful not to stretch to your extreme. Stretch

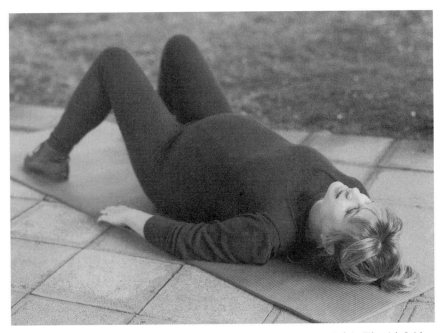

Pelvic Tilt with Bridge

The Test for Diastasis Recti

Lie on your back with your knees bent and your feet flat on the floor. Place your fingertips just above or below your navel. Lift your head and shoulders off the floor and pull your chin to your chest. This will feel like you're doing an abdominal curl. Now press down firmly and feel for any separation between the bands of vertical muscles. If the separation is greater than two fingers wide, you've probably got diastasis recti.

If you do, you should use a splint when you do abdominal work. Kathy used a neoprene waistband that fastened across her abs with velcro. It cost about $20 in a sporting-goods store. Or you can take a long strip of material—a sturdy scarf works well—and, when you're on the floor, put the scarf under your back and pull the ends around your middle. Hold each end with the opposite hand and pull tight. You're pulling your two long muscles together. Hold them together as you do your abdominal curls. This will help to strengthen those weakened muscles.

slowly and carefully, paying attention to what your body is telling you.

And right now, we're telling your body to take a break and relax. (After you've finished, have something nutritious to eat. Your body needs 300 extra calories a day when you are pregnant.)

You've completed a week of workouts. You're sure to get good reviews from all your admirers. Congratulations!

You can continue these three workouts (Monday, Wednesday, and Friday) throughout your entire pregnancy. Modify any of the moves if it will make you feel more comfortable. Try to perform at top level, though, because you will find it will make a big difference in delivery and beyond.

We know because it has worked for us.

Warning Signs*

If you get any of these symptoms and they are unusually severe, stop exercising and contact your doctor immediately:

- Pain
- Dizziness
- Shortness of breath
- Feeling faint
- Vaginal bleeding
- Rapid heartbeat while resting
- Difficulty walking
- Contractions of the uterus
- No fetal movements

*Source: ACOG (The American College of Obstetricians and Gynecologists)

WARM-UP SUMMARY

EXERCISE	REPS	SETS
March in Place	10	3
Side Step/Lateral Arm Raise	10	3
Alternate Legs Back/Swing Arms	10	3
Shoulder Roll	10	1

COOL-DOWN SUMMARY

EXERCISE	REPS	SETS
Arm-Leg Opposition		
right	hold 10 to 30 seconds	1
left	hold 10 to 30 seconds	1
V-Sit Stretch		
right	hold 10 to 30 seconds	1
left	hold 10 to 30 seconds	1
Butterfly Stretch	hold 10 to 30 seconds	1
Cat Stretch		
round up back	6 to 8	1
squat position—arm stretch	hold 10 to 30 seconds	1
squat position—arms at sides	hold as long as possible	1
round up back	6 to 8	1

PREGNANCY WORKOUT
MONDAY SUMMARY*

EXERCISE	REPS	SETS
Overhead Press	8	1
Sit-Down Squat	10	1
Reverse Fly	8	1
Side Leg Lift		
right	15	1
left	15	1
Pelvic Tilt	25	1
Kegel	25	1
Accordion	25 exhales	1

* Repeat exercises or add sets at your discretion.

PREGNANCY WORKOUT
WEDNESDAY SUMMARY*

EXERCISE	REPS	SETS
Plié Squat	10	1
Military Press	8	1
Split Lunge		
right	10	1
left	10	1
Lateral Raise	8	1
Shoulder Press (3-Count Press)	10	1
Pelvic Tilt with Bridge	25	1
Kegel	25	1
Abdominal Curl	25	1
Accordion	25 exhales	1

* Repeat exercises or add sets at your discretion.

PREGNANCY WORKOUT
FRIDAY SUMMARY*

EXERCISE	REPS	SETS
Plié Leg Lift		
right	10	1
left	10	1
Triceps Dip	10	1
Standing Side Leg Lift		
right	15	1
left	15	1
Biceps Curl	10	1
Seated Row	15	1
Push-Up	10	1
Kegel	25	1
Pelvic Tilt with Bridge	25	1
Accordion	25 exhales	1

* Repeat exercises or add sets at your discretion.

TWO

High Anxiety

Pregnancy—Your Last Months

No matter how much an actor loves playing a particular role, there comes a time when she feels like she has exhausted the challenge of the character she's playing and is ready to find a new vehicle for her talents.

If you're in the last months of your pregnancy, you are probably feeling the same way. It's not that you don't love walking around feeling special as the nurturer of that new little life inside you, it's just that you'd like to walk into a room first, *before* your belly gets there. And while your enlarged breasts may be the object of enlarged affection, you're the one with the backaches from schlepping around those heavy, bloated glands on your chest.

And let's not forget the high anxiety you're feeling about . . . well, just about everything. You want to get through all that hard "labor" of labor. You want to hold that baby in your arms instead of your belly. You want the reality of seeing that it's a healthy baby. And you want your body back—not only where it was before you got pregnant but better and stronger. Wouldn't it be nice to be admired for your shapely body instead of your round shape?

Until the baby arrives, the only thing you'll be able to shape up is your attitude because basically the grand Mother of us all, Mother Nature, will be dictating just about everything else to you.

If you're like most people, by your second trimester, your hormones have redesigned your body. Your butt and your thighs are wider and rounder, and your upper arms and shoulders have pads of fat around them. Your face puffs up and so do your hands and feet.

Kathy, who ultimately gained 73 pounds in her pregnancy, stopped wearing regular shoes in her sixth month, resorting to clogs and sandals; her wedding ring came off when she was five months pregnant (and didn't get back on until six months after the twins were born); and her face was so swollen that her bloated tongue kept her from being able to close her mouth.

All the time that her body grew beyond her control, her emotions did, too. Never given to mood swings before, she found herself alternately anxious, fearful, and depressed. As a college student, Kathy was bulimic, and those old fears of loss of control over her body were trying to take over. Somewhere in the latter part of her second trimester, she

realized she had to disengage herself emotionally from the weight gain her body was experiencing. She came to accept the fact that her growth in size was a necessary condition for nurturing the babies. Then there was the supreme disengagement for Kathy when she was five months pregnant: Her doctor told her that if she wanted to continue working, she had to stop exercising.

By her eighth and ninth months when she could barely see her feet, which were huge, when none of her oversized clothing fit, when she looked in the mirror and couldn't even detect cheekbones, she decided to give in and indulge. She ate ice cream, popcorn, and candy at the movies.

Of course, there's a happy ending to Kathy's story: her two healthy, beautiful baby boys and a body that looks fabulous.

While most women have some measure of the body changes that Kathy had in her pregnancy, not every woman's body handles her hormones as dramatically as Kathy's did.

Meg Ryan is a case in point. Meg was already pregnant when she started working out with Kathy. Meg had been physically active before she met Kathy, so when the two of them started training, Kathy felt Meg was capable of doing a pretty hardy aerobic workout along with body shaping and strengthening. Meg alternated between step aerobics and hiking every other day for 45 minutes to 1 hour each session.

When she did step, she worked with 2-pound hand weights, and when she hiked, she hiked up and down hills. And, as we've been urging you to do, Kathy made sure to work with Meg on her upper-body strength. She concentrated on biceps curls, lateral raises, and overhead presses.

As her pregnancy progressed, Meg slowed down her speed and Kathy decreased Meg's amount of time on the step from 45 minutes to 35 minutes to 25 minutes. Because they were afraid of tripping or falling while hiking, they eliminated the outdoor work. As for the upper-body work, they continued to do it all, but with fewer repetitions.

Meg, who is naturally quite lean, did not have to deal with any real swelling during her pregnancy. She gained about 19 pounds total and she worked out until the day she gave birth.

Michelle Pfeiffer worked out until one week before she gave birth. Michelle, who had started training with Kathy in order to get into shape for the role of Catwoman in *Batman Returns*, was very fit before she got pregnant. She had been running four to five miles a day two times a week. Soon after she became pregnant, she cut down on the number of days she ran by half and she cut the number of miles from five to three. She alternated her running with low-impact aerobics.

In Michelle's fourth month of pregnancy, her body started sending her signals that caused Kathy to readjust Michelle's workout. They went from running to walking outside or on the treadmill. By slowing down to a walk, they took away the impact and intensity while maintaining the cardio benefits. In Michelle's gym, they cross trained with the stationary bike, the treadmill, and the step.

When she started to feel light-headed while stepping, they slowed down the tempo of the music and took away one step so Michelle could exert less energy on the lift.

She continued to exercise five days a week, for an hour each day. Remember, from the time she was three months pregnant until she was seven months pregnant, Michelle was shooting a major motion picture (*Dangerous Minds*), which had her in practically every single scene. She had great endurance.

Despite her enlarged size and

her heavy work schedule, Michelle did some form of exercise throughout her pregnancy. Her last workout was a week before she delivered. Kathy and Michelle starting walking from Michelle's house on a hot August morning. After about eight to ten minutes, the heat and her weight combined to slow her down so much that Michelle went back home and, just like Kathy did at the end of her pregnancy, she relaxed and waited for her baby to arrive.

Jami Gertz kept exercising throughout both of her two pregnancies. She was fit before she became pregnant each time and she gained 35 pounds with each baby (they were two years and ten months apart).

During her first pregnancy, Jami did step aerobics and during her second pregnancy she walked on the treadmill and did weight training. She also did the muscle shaping and strengthening exercises we have scripted for you.

While Jami tried to keep her workouts as smooth in schedule and frequency as possible, there were some obstacles. There were the vomiting spells we told you about in Chapter 1 and there was the breathlessness.

Let's take a moment here to address that breathless feeling so many pregnant women complain of having. Kathy felt it period-ically early in her pregnancy and almost all the time by the end.

This shortness of breath is not atypical by the second trimester. As the uterus grows, it moves the diaphragm upward so that when you breathe, your diaphragm's movement is restricted. Since the diaphragm separates the lungs from the abdominal cavity and helps regulate breathing, when its movement is restricted, it feels like you can't breathe deeply enough, especially when you're trying to take in more oxygen during exercise.

Don't be alarmed over this feeling. Instead exhale slowly then inhale slowly. Relax, inhale, and exhale again. You should feel fine enough to continue on with what you were doing. During your pregnancy, especially as the end comes closer, when you exercise, remember to work at a tempo and intensity that doesn't make you feel breathless. Keep in mind the rule we gave you in the last chapter: You should be able to string together four words without gulping for air. The idea behind exercising throughout your pregnancy is to feel better; it's not about burning fat. You've got to let your body do its job.

While Jami had to curtail the intensity of her workouts, she never gave up on them because exercising made her feel stronger.

Even at the end, when she couldn't see her toes and she found herself stuck between two exercise machines in the gym as she tried to waddle between them, all she could think about was getting back into her familiar old jeans, so she kept going.

And so can you. Follow our *Primetime Pregnancy* workout in Chapter 1. Even though you may be feeling that high anxiety over changing roles from "almost mom" to mom, you still need a little more preparation for your new role. And doing however much or little exercise you can will help. You're just like an actress performing in front of the camera. Though the script and the director guide you, the quality of your performance is up to you.

Michelle, Meg, and Jami had the same script you do. Their director, Kathy, is your director.

The rest is up to you. We think you can do it. Good luck and we'll see you after the baby is born.

A Note About Your Progressing Pregnancy

We've given you a few exercises that call for you to lie on your back. They are

- Pelvic Tilt
- Pelvic Tilt with Bridge
- Abdominal Curl
- Kegel

Each one of these moves, with the number of repetitions we have called for, should take no more than a minute to do. That is a limited enough amount of time that you should be able to do these exercises throughout your entire pregnancy.

For some of you, by the time you get into your second trimester, you may find lying on your back difficult. That's because, in this position, your enlarged uterus puts some pressure on the vein that returns blood to the heart. This pressure could make you feel dizzy or nauseated. If you do feel those symptoms, gently roll onto your left side.

You can do the pelvic tilt standing up against the wall (see page 47). You will probably have to give up doing the pelvic tilt with bridge if lying on your back is uncomfortable for you.

You can substitute what we call the side-lying abdominal curl for the regular abdominal curl. Lying on your side, hold the back of your head with your hands. Bend your knees at a 45-degree

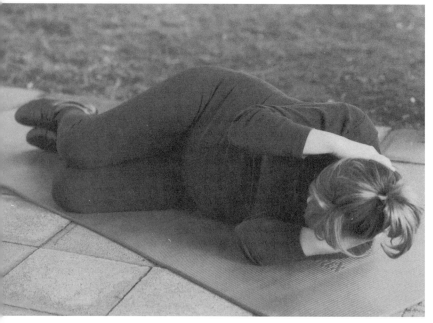

Side-Lying Abdominal Curl

angle to your hips. Your knees and hips are stacked. Now bring your knees up toward your chest. Exhale as you bring your head and shoulders down toward your bent knees and inhale as you straighten your upper body.

Do whatever number of reps is called for in that day's workout.

You can also do the kegels on your side (see page 24 for kegels description).

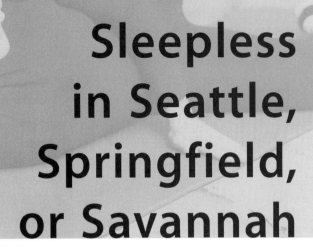

Sleepless in Seattle, Springfield, or Savannah

Three

Your First Postpregnancy Month

*L*et's face it, your body has just gone through a major assault. And now that the baby is out, you want to reclaim your pre-pregnancy body—immediately! But your combat wounds are still sore; the baby doesn't know the difference between night and day so you can't get any decent sleep; and, to top it all off, you're feeling those "postpartum blues," which leave you anxious and lonely. In short, this is not the greatest time of your life . . . and yet it is.

The first few weeks after the baby is born, you're making many big adjustments, both physically and emotionally. You're bonding with your baby and you're basking in the accomplishment of having given birth. Now, after nine months of your catching the spotlight, the spotlight is shining on your creation. A star is born and you're the center of her universe.

It almost makes you want to forget about what your mirror is reflecting: stretched muscles and loose skin. In fact, you look like you're six months pregnant. Don't feel bad. You're not alone. When she got pregnant, Kathy weighed 145 pounds and had a body composition of 11 percent fat (acceptable range is 16 to 22 percent body fat for women and most American women have 25 to 35 percent body fat). When she went into the hospital to deliver Cooper and Payton, Kathy weighed 218 pounds. The day she left, she weighed 191 pounds, and two weeks later, she weighed in at 188 pounds, which was what Kathy weighed when she was six months pregnant!

Many women lose 15 to 20 pounds within a couple of weeks after giving birth. When Michelle left the hospital a couple of days after her son was born, she had shed 20 of her 28 pounds. The initial weight loss is due to the weight of the baby and a pound or two of placenta and amniotic fluid. But it usually takes a month or two for your blood and hormone levels to get back to normal, so your body holds on to the fat deposits as if it were still in a pregnant state.

And then there is breast-feeding. For some women, breast-feeding helps them lose weight faster. Michelle lost a pound a day when she breast-fed. Most women hold on to at least an extra five pounds while they breast-feed because they need extra nourishment to keep their milk flowing steadily.

A nursing mother needs to eat an extra 500 calories a day above what she was consuming pre-pregnancy. Some women need fewer calories because their bodies have extra fat stored and that fat gets burned to produce milk. Women who are underweight will need more than 500 calories to help them nurse.

Some women use the fact that they are breast-feeding to indulge in foods that they might otherwise not eat. Michelle did. She had a baby nurse who kept a watchful eye over her and who didn't let her overindulge in cakes and cookies, but she did have a lot of fun eating more than usual. But then, Michelle was losing weight anyway.

Rita Wilson was a different story. In good shape before she got pregnant and exercising throughout her pregnancy, Rita gained just 12 pounds with her first baby and 16 pounds with her second. After the birth of each baby she was in pretty good shape, but gradually she gained weight while she was nursing. Within six months after giving birth, she had gained up to about ten extra pounds (ice cream was her weakness!).

So here is a case of a woman who was fit before getting pregnant, remained fit during pregnancy, and gained very little weight; yet six months after the babies were born—a time when most women have achieved or are close to achieving their pre-pregnancy weight—Rita was on the phone asking Kathy for extra help.

Nine months after her second child was born, Rita got a role in the movie *Jingle All the Way* with Arnold Schwarzenegger. Her part called for her to wear a silk negligee, and there was no way she wanted that extra weight around her middle showing through. So Kathy put her through many of the same exercises you'll be doing in the next five months as you follow the routines in *Primetime Pregnancy*.

The key to starting your post-pregnancy exercising is to start slowly. Some women exercise the day after they give birth, other women rest. If it doesn't feel good, wait. But if you feel up to any working out, do not include aerobics. Your joints are still too loose and prone to injury. If you had an episiotomy, you want to be careful about loosening the stitches, and if you had a cesarean section, you're required to rest for three to six weeks before resuming exercise.

For the first month (at least) after the baby is born, your schedule will be topsy turvy. So we suggest splitting up the different exercises we have scripted for you to do at different times during the day or night. You can do the exercises between feedings, naps, and eating. For instance, you can do kegels in the morning and accordions at noon. You need to promote strength in these two areas that have been weakened by pregnancy and birth. Then in the evening you can do shoulder circles and the neck releases to help loosen your shoulders and upper back from the tensions of the day.

Postpregnancy Workout—Weeks 1 and 2

Kegel

You can do these sitting, standing, or on your back before you get out of bed in the morning.

If you do them on your back, your knees are bent and your feet are flat on the floor. Your hands are by your sides and your head and neck can be resting on your pillow.

Now squeeze the PC muscle. Hold the squeeze for 1 second and release. Now repeat the squeeze and hold.

Do this 30 times these first couple of weeks.

Pelvic Tilt Against Wall

Try doing these pelvic tilts while you're leaning against a wall. It will help your posture as well as help you strengthen your pelvic floor and your abs.

Put your back straight up against the wall. Your heels are as close to the wall as possible. Your hands are down at your sides. Inhale while you press the small of your back against the wall, tilting your pelvis forward. Now exhale and release.

Count each inhale and release as 1 rep. Do 10 reps.

Accordion

Remember, the key to the accordion is to expand your abs on the inhale and pull them in on the exhale.

Stand with your knees slightly bent and your pelvis tilted slightly forward. Take a deep breath in, filling your belly to expand your accordion fully. Now exhale, pulling in until the accordion is halfway closed. The exercise really starts here where the accordion is half closed. You exhale further and blow all the air out to close it.

Each halfway closure to complete closure is 1 rep. Count out loud every time you pull back toward your spine. Here's the rhythm: inhale, exhale, small rhythmic exhales with small contractions.

Count each of these smaller exhales as 1 rep. Do 15 reps.

Shoulder Circle

You can do these any time of the day, but by the end of the day, they're mandatory. Your shoulders and upper back may still be aching from the tension during labor. And you're probably feeling soreness from lifting the baby and breast-feeding. By the end of the day you could use some relief and these shoulder circles will help alleviate upper-body soreness.

Stand with your feet a few inches apart and your arms down at your sides. Your knees are relaxed. Now gently lift your shoulders up toward your ears and roll your shoulders back, squeezing your shoulder blades together and down. Reverse the move so that your arms and shoulders circle back up and forward toward your ears. Lower your shoulders.

Count each circle back, down, up, and forward as 1 rep. Do 8 reps.

Neck Release

Stand in the same basic position as you did for the shoulder circles. Your feet are slightly apart and your knees are soft—not locked into place. Your arms are down at your sides.

Tilt your head to your right so that your right ear aims down toward your right shoulder. Do not lift your shoulder and do not force

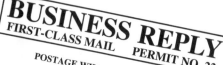

If you can, do these exercises
throughout your first two
postpartum weeks, and you'll start
to build some strength as your
body heals from the trauma of
labor and delivery.

If you're feeling strong
enough in these two weeks, and
you're not bleeding, an easy walk
around the block is a good idea to
get your heart and lungs going.

Postpregnancy Workout—Weeks 3 and 4

By the third and fourth weeks
after the baby is born, you can
increase the intensity of your
workout. The kegels you've been

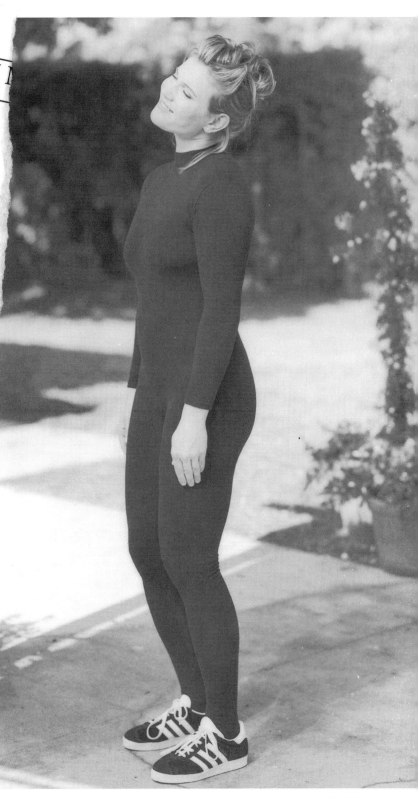

Neck Release

doing have helped heal the area around the episiotomy so you should now be able to increase the repetitions. Your abs and pelvic floor continue to need your attention, as does your upper back. These areas, which were under the most stress throughout your pregnancy, need extra attention as you work on getting back into shape.

You can do the exercises we have scripted for weeks 3 and 4 as a complete routine that should take you about 15 minutes from warm-up to cool-down. If you can't find that chunk of time, divide up the routine and do different exercises as time becomes available.

If you're feeling up to it, walk for 15 or 20 minutes at least three times a week. Then, follow your walk with our routine. If you can only do our workout, our warm-up will get your heart and lungs into workout mode. You can continue to use our pre-pregnancy warm-up. It's on page 7.

If going through the warm-up one time leaves you feeling sufficiently energized, start your workout. If you want to, repeat the entire warm-up and then start the workout that we've designed for your third and fourth post-pregnancy weeks.

PROPS

- Hand weights
- Straight-back chair
- Doughnut

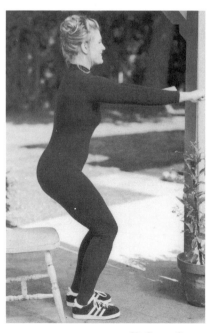 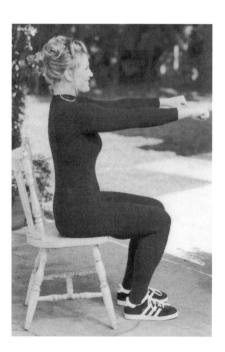

Sit-Down Squat

Rear Deltoid Squeeze

Stand with your feet shoulder-width apart. Your pelvis is in a neutral position. Rotate your shoulder blades back and squeeze them together. Hold this position for 8 to 10 seconds and then release.

Sit-Down Squat

Stand with your back to the seat of your chair. You should be about two feet away from the chair. Now, as if you were going to sit on the chair, lower your butt and upper body toward the chair. Lower your butt to the chair seat and, keeping your weight on your heels, lift back to the standing position. Use your arms to balance you as you move down and up. Do not use your arms to push yourself up.

If you had an episiotomy and this tapping on the chair is uncomfortable, put a doughnut on the chair.

Count each sit down and lift as 1 rep. Do 10 reps.

Accordion

This time we'll try the accordions on your hands and knees. Your back should not be arched. It should be straight. Visualize the accordion attached to your spine and hanging down toward the floor. Take a deep breath in through your belly. This will fill your accordion so it fully expands.

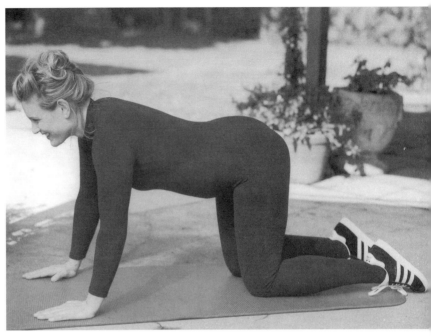

Accordion

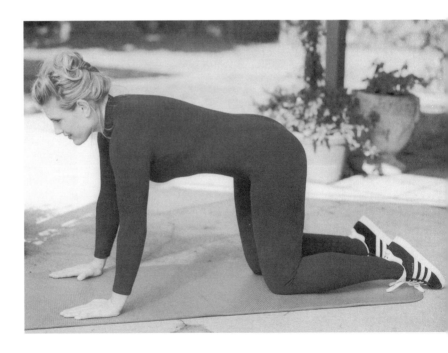

Exhale and pull in until your accordion closes halfway. Then fill and empty the accordion from halfway closed to closed, counting each short, rhythmic exhale/inhale as 1 rep. Do 20 reps.

Pelvic Tilt with Bridge

Come down onto your back. Your head and shoulders rest comfortably on the floor. Bend your knees. Now, squeezing your lower abs and gluts, tilt your pelvis up so that your gluts lift off the floor. Squeeze higher (the bridge) so that your lower back comes up off the floor. Hold for 1 second then lower your butt back onto the floor. Each lift and lower is 1 rep.

Do 20 reps.

While you're working your pelvic floor, you're strengthening your gluts, quads, and hamstrings.

Side Leg Lift

Turn onto your left side. Start with your body in a straight line so that your left arm extends straight as do your legs. Keep your hips stacked as you bend your knees so they're between 45 and 90 degrees from your upper body. The inside of your right knee mirrors the inside of your left knee. Flex your right foot.

Bend your left arm and lift your head, resting it on your left hand. Place your right arm in front

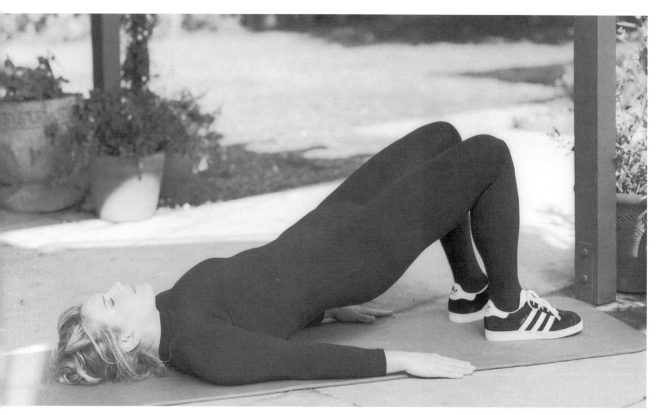

Pelvic Tilt with Bridge

of you, fixing it firmly so you don't rock back as you lift your right leg. Feel that tension in the outer thigh and hip as you lift against gravity?

Now bring down the right leg, squeezing your gluts and inner thigh muscles as if you had a ball between your knees. You can even tighten your PC muscle and do a kegel at the same time. Don't let your upper leg rest, lift it again.

Count each lift and lower as 1 rep. Do 15 reps.

Now turn over onto your right side and repeat this move with your left leg. Your hips are stacked and your knees are bent. Flex your left foot and place your left arm in front of you as an anchor. Rest your head on your right hand. Now, keeping your upper body steady, lift your left leg against gravity. Then lower it, squeezing down and squeezing your gluts. Do 15 reps. Stay right where you are for your kegels.

Kegel

Stay on your right side, with your knees bent, your legs stacked on top of each other, and your head resting on your right arm. Now, squeeze and hold that PC muscle. Hold it for 1 second and then release it.

Do 50 of these kegels.

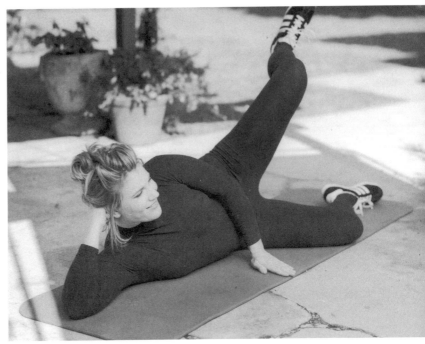

Side Leg Lift

If you're up to it, go back and repeat the entire circuit. If you want to isolate one or two of the exercises for repetition, feel free to do so. If you feel you've done enough for today, please turn to our cool-down on page 16.

Do this entire routine at least three times a week. You'll soon start to feel the results of your efforts and it won't take long until you start to see those results, too.

In the meantime, sticking to a regular workout says a lot about you. You're on your way toward turning a dream into a reality and that's the stuff good scripts are made of!

POSTPREGNANCY WORKOUT
WEEKS 1 AND 2 SUMMARY*

EXERCISE	REPS	SETS
Kegel	30	1
Pelvic Tilt Against Wall	10	1
Accordion	15 exhales	1
Shoulder Circle	8	1
Neck Release		
right	hold 15 seconds	1
left	hold 15 seconds	1

* If you feel strong enough, repeat exercises or add sets at your discretion.

POSTPREGNANCY WORKOUT
WEEKS 3 AND 4 SUMMARY*

EXERCISE	REPS	SETS
Rear Deltoid Squeeze	hold 8 to 10 seconds	1
Sit-Down Squat	10	1
Accordion	20 exhales	1
Pelvic Tilt with Bridge	20	1
Side Leg Lift		
right	15	1
left	15	1
Kegel	50	1

* If you feel strong enough, repeat exercises or add sets at your
discretion.

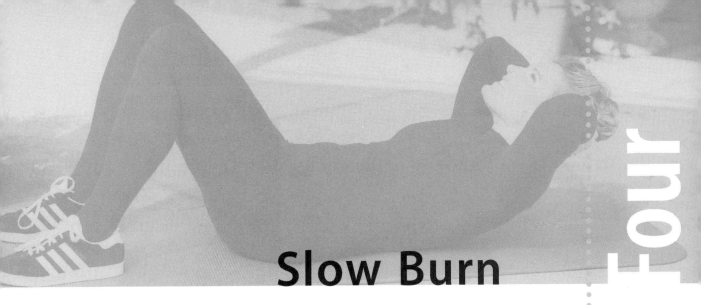

Four

Slow Burn

Month 2: Basic Cardio and Toning

Meg Ryan and Rita Wilson both gained fewer than 20 pounds in their pregnancies. Kathy gained more than 70 pounds. Chances are you're somewhere in between with the amount of weight you gained.

Meg started walking around the golf course with her husband, Dennis Quaid, about two and a half weeks after her baby was born. He may have only played nine holes but that translates into two hours of outdoor activity. Kathy could barely do ten minutes on the recumbent bike when she was three weeks postpartum.

The point we're trying to make is that every woman's body reacts differently to pregnancy and to postpregnancy. Every woman should listen to what her body is telling her, especially when it comes to exercise, and act accordingly.

We believe that, starting with the second month after the baby is born, it's a good idea for you to begin making at least 20 minutes of aerobic activity an integral part of your day. Stimulating your cardiovascular system for 20 minutes is a good way to initiate your fat-burning program, and that 20 minutes will help boost your energy level. As you're discovering, your new baby and everything that she or he demands means extra energy is a necessity. Another great by-product of exercise is that it works as a mood elevator.

This second month, most likely, you're still feeling very attached to your baby, and you don't want to separate yourself from him or her for very long. We think you can include the baby in your workout starting with a 20-minute walk in the mall, pushing the baby in the stroller.

Shoot for a 20-minute mile or walk 20 or even 30 minutes without stopping. Make sure your breathing has increased and you feel slight perspiration on your skin. With a good exercise walk, you'll feel a contraction in your leg muscles.

You can also do low-intensity aerobics and have the baby in the room with you. Or you can do indoor bicycling—preferably on a recumbent bike because it supports your lower back. Whatever exercise you choose, be careful about any sudden or strenuous movements because your muscles and ligaments are still loose from your raised hormonal level.

Postpregnancy Workout—Month 2

After you've done your 20-minute workout, try our muscle strengthening and shaping routine. We've included the baby in these exercises. You can hold him or her close and use baby's body weight as resistance. Your baby should enjoy the movement as well as the bonding he or she will feel with you.

Unless you've just completed your aerobics and your muscles are still warm, start with our warm-up and then go right into the routine we have scripted for this month. If you're looking for variety or to increase the workload, feel free to borrow any of the moves from last month.

Of course, anytime we ask you to work with the baby in an exercise and you don't find that comfortable, you can certainly do the exercise alone and, where appropriate, you can use hand weights.

First, turn to page 7 for our warm-up, and then start the routine.

PROPS

- Straight-back chair
- Hand weights
- Your baby

Plié with Baby

Hold your baby in your arms so that he or she is fully supported. Baby's body should be vertical, with back against your chest. Stand with your legs more than shoulder-width apart. If there were a clock under you, your toes would be pointed in the ten o'clock and two o'clock positions.

Bend your knees and lower your body so that your torso comes down toward the floor. As you get deeper into your bend, your knees come over your toes but your torso remains upright. Do not let your butt go any lower than your knees. Your knees should be at a 45-degree angle to your ankles.

Now lift up, squeezing your gluts. You'll feel the resistance from your baby's weight as you lift. Stop when your knees are slightly bent. You don't want to straighten your legs because you want to keep the tension in your inner thighs.

Count each plié down and the lift up as 1 rep. Do 10 reps.

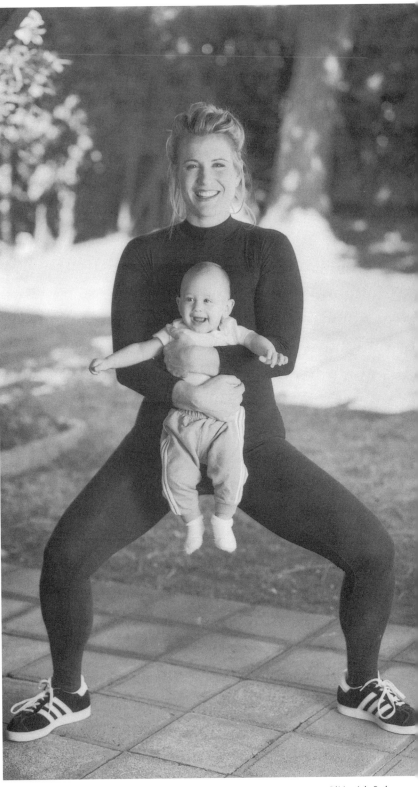

Plié with Baby

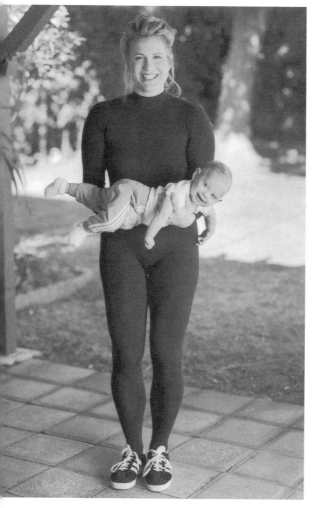
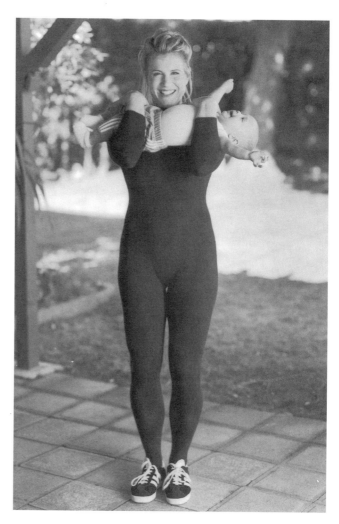

Biceps Curl with Baby

Biceps Curl with Baby

Hold your baby so his or her body is lengthwise across your chest and is resting on your forearms. Baby's head is supported by one of your arms and the bottom part of his or her body with your other arm. Your elbows are bent and they are at your sides, waist high.

Stand with your feet shoulder-width apart. This time your toes are facing forward. Your knees are slightly bent.

Now curl your arms up so that your baby comes in toward your chest. Lower your forearms so your baby goes back to the waist-high starting position.

Count each curl up and down as 1 rep. Do 10 reps.

Put baby in his or her swing or chair so baby can watch you do the next five exercises.

Plié with Side Leg Lift

Take your chair and stand facing the back of the chair. Hold on to it lightly for balance. Put your feet in the ten o'clock and two o'clock positions, and your legs are more than shoulder-width apart. Lower with your torso straight so your butt comes down toward the floor and your knees come out over your toes. Do not let your butt go any lower than your knees, and then lift.

When you get to the top, do not lock your knees. Keep them soft. Now with the toes of your right foot pointed forward, lift your right leg out and away from your left leg. Keep your right leg straight as it pushes against your right hip. You will not be able to lift your right leg very high. Try and keep your body as straight as you can, without leaning over to the left side. Now lower your leg and put your right foot back into the plié position. And get ready to repeat.

Count this plié, lift, and side leg lift as 1 rep. Do 5 reps.

Now lower into another plié and then lift. This time turn the toes of your left leg forward and lift your left leg out to the side and away from the standing leg. Return the left leg to the plié position and lower into another plié.

Do 5 reps—plié, lift, and side leg lift—with your left leg.

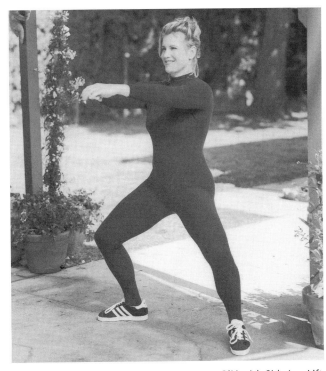
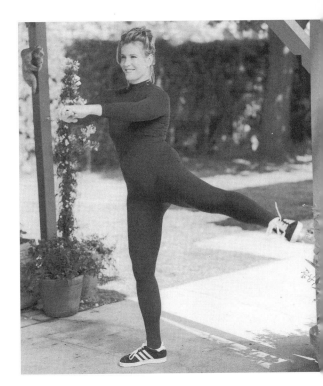

Plié with Side Leg Lift

Overhead Press

Stand in the basic position with your legs apart and your knees slightly bent. Your pelvis is neutral—it does not tilt forward or backward.

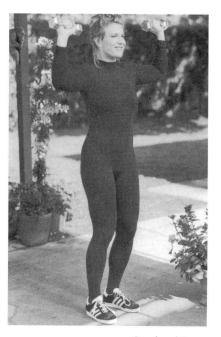

Overhead Press

Take a weight in each hand. You start with your arms bent at the elbow and lifted so that your hands are parallel with the tops of your shoulders. Your hands are facing forward.

Press your arms up overhead. Exhale as you lift. Your arms are fully extended overhead and you hold for a beat, then inhale as you return your arms to their original position. Repeat.

Count each press overhead and return to the original position as 1 rep. Do 15 reps.

Triceps Dip

We women have a tendency to carry weight in our upper arms, and when you were pregnant you probably noticed that extra fat pad in that area. It's not an easy area to whip into shape but triceps dips are an effective way to target your upper arms.

Start by sitting on the very edge of the chair with your knees bent in front of you. Put your arms behind you with the heels of your palms on the edge of the chair. Now take your butt off the chair as you bend your elbows and dip so your bottom and your back skim the chair seat as you lower. Do not touch the floor with your butt. Exhale and lift back up. Repeat.

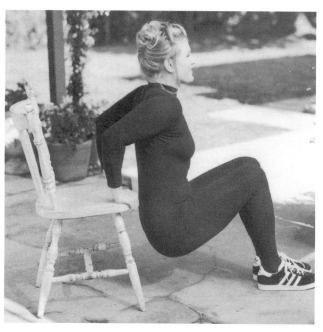

Triceps Dip

Count each dip and lift as 1 rep. Do 10 reps. The backs of your arms will really feel these.

Seated Row

We'll keep working your arms, upper back, and shoulders with this one. You need to continue to pay special attention to these areas because of the constant strain they get from lifting the baby and from holding the baby in the nursing or feeding position.

Get down on the floor with your exercise band, old panty hose, or tights. Your legs, extended in front of you, are about hip-width apart. As usual, your knees are slightly bent. Wrap the band or hose around the bottom of your feet. Hold each end of the flexible material so that your palms face inward toward your body. Depending on the length you may have to wrap the band or hose around your hands. In their unstretched position the band or the hose should come up to mid-calf.

Your back should be straight but bent slightly forward at the waist as you grasp the ends of the material. Flex your feet and pull the material backward as you exhale. Your elbows bend as you pull the material. You pull in on your abs and bring your upper body into a straight position as the material becomes taut in your hands, and you feel the tension of the pull in your upper arms, shoulders, and upper back.

Release your arms so that they're extended forward. Keep your back straight. Now repeat the rowing motion from this straight back position. Your elbows will bend as you pull your fist back toward your rib cage.

Count each row back and release as 1 rep. Do 15 reps.

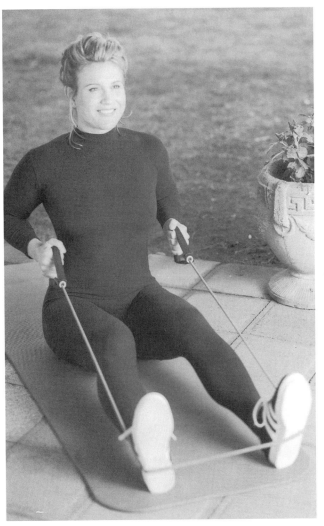

Seated Row

Side Leg Lift

You stay on the floor and come onto your right side. Extend your right arm. Your hips are stacked, your legs are together, and your knees are slightly bent—between 45 and 90 degrees. Bend your right arm at the elbow and rest your head on your right hand.

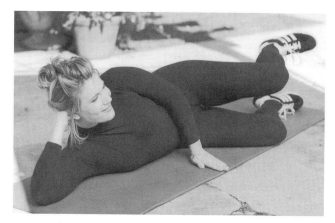

Side Leg Lift

Place your left arm in front of you as an anchor so you don't move your upper body.

Flex your left foot and lift your leg up so that your knee comes just a little higher than hip level. (You can't lift much higher if you don't tilt backward.) Now lower your leg but don't rest it on your right leg; instead lift again.

Count each lift and lowering of the leg as 1 rep. Do 20 reps and then switch sides.

Now on your left side, extend your left arm. Your hips are stacked and your legs are together with your knees slightly bent. Bend your left arm at the elbow and rest your head on your left hand. Your right arm is your anchor.

Flex your right foot and lift your leg so that your knee lifts a little higher than hip level. Now lower your leg without resting it. Lift it again.

Do 20 reps.

Chest Press with Baby

It's time to bring baby back into the act. So bring baby onto the floor. Lie down while you're holding the baby under his or her arms, perpendicular to you and facing you. Bend your knees slightly and sit the baby on your abs. Lift the baby up without lifting your head, neck, or shoulders off the floor. Hold the

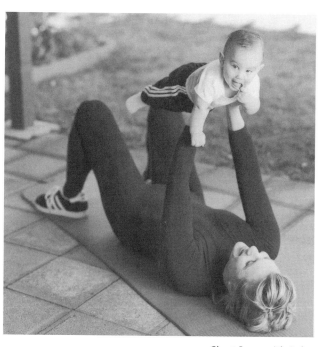

Chest Press with Baby

baby up for a beat and then lower him or her back onto your abs.

Count each lift, hold, and lower as 1 rep. Do 10 reps.

This exercise should be a lot of fun for both you and your baby.

Pelvic Tilt with Bridge and Baby

Stay in the same position. Bring your knees up a little higher by bringing your heels an inch or two closer to your butt. Rest the baby against your quads while he or she sits on your abs. Hold baby in place facing you.

Now tilt your pelvis up so that your butt squeezes up off the floor. Your abs tighten as you exhale. Your lower back comes slightly off the floor. The baby's weight is adding resistance. Keep squeezing your butt and holding your lower back off the floor. Hold for a beat and lower.

Count each pelvic tilt and lower as 1 rep. Do 10 reps. Rest about 5 seconds and do a second set of 10.

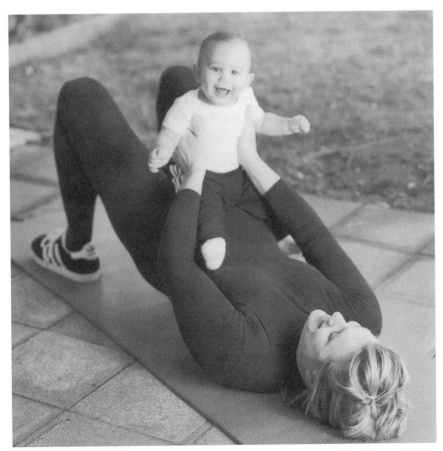

Pelvic Tilt with Bridge and Baby

Accordion

Baby gets to play the accordion with you, too! You're still on the floor and your knees are still bent. The baby remains sitting on your lower abs. Now take a deep breath in through your belly, expanding that imaginary accordion. Exhale so you close the accordion, bringing your belly in halfway toward your spine.

In the half-closed position, take a series of short, rhythmic breaths, blowing out and counting as you go from halfway to totally closed on each exhale. Count 50 of these short breaths out loud to your baby.

Crunch with Pelvic Tilt

Let baby watch you do these. Remain on your back. Clasp your hands behind your head for support. Your knees are bent, and your feet are flat on the floor. Tilt your pelvis as you lift your upper body toward your bent knees. Imagine your bottom rib and your hip bones coming closer together as you move. (You can squeeze your PC muscle here, too, getting a head start on the kegels, which

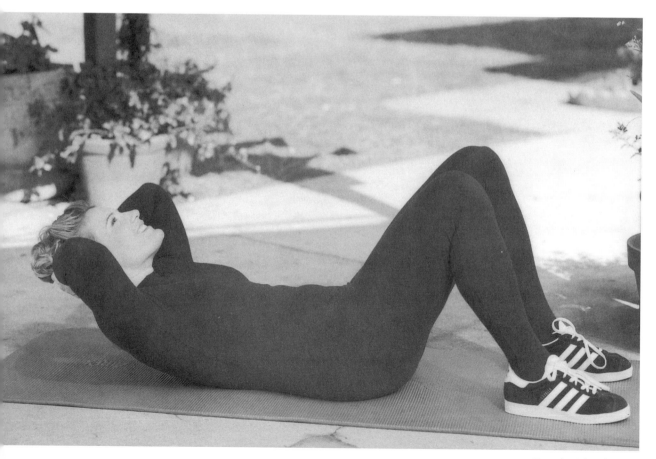

Crunch with Pelvic Tilt

come next.) Lower your shoulders but don't rest at the bottom.

Do 20 reps.

Kegel

You can stay right where you are but bring your hands down at your sides. Now, without moving any other part of your body, squeeze your pubo-coccygeal (PC) muscle. Remember, it feels as if you're holding back a flow of urine. Hold the squeeze for 1 second. Count out loud. Release and repeat.

Do 50 of these kegels. You're still working on tightening up that area and it's going to take a while to get it back into pre-pregnancy shape. The good news is that the more you work on strengthening this muscle, the better chance you have of making it stronger than it

ever was. And that's our intention for you throughout the next months. We want to make you stronger than you were before baby came along. And we can do it—with your help. We're like an ensemble theater group. The more we perform the script together, the stronger and better our performance.

Follow our script all this month, three to five performances a week. If you don't have time to do the entire circuit at once, do a matinee and an evening performance, dividing the workout in half. The important thing is to just do it. We know you can.

As for today's performance, remember: it's not complete until you do the cool-down on page 16.

POSTPREGNANCY WORKOUT
MONTH 2 SUMMARY*

EXERCISE	REPS	SETS
Plié with Baby	10	1
Biceps Curl with Baby	10	1
Plié with Side Leg Lift		
right	5	1
left	5	1
Overhead Press	15	1
Triceps Dip	10	1
Seated Row	15	1
Side Leg Lift		
right	20	1
left	20	1
Chest Press with Baby	10	1
Pelvic Tilt with Bridge and Baby	10	2
Accordion	50 exhales	1
Crunch with Pelvic Tilt	20	1
Kegel	50	1

* Repeat exercises or add sets at your discretion.

Stand and Deliver

Five

Month 3:
Adding Time and Intensity

*W*e're going to make it harder on you this month by adding repetitions and intensity. By now you should be stronger and, we hope, the weight has been coming off steadily. This is the month when your body is telling you it's ready to push harder and you can go back to your pre-pregnancy workout level. You can push yourself to a 15-minute mile on the treadmill; you can do 40 minutes of aerobics and you can even add impact to your moves. You can add swimming to your choices of aerobic activity without running the risk of infection.

But remember, everyone is different. At three months postpartum, Kathy was still feeling soreness around her incision, while Jami Gertz was getting ready to take off and shoot the hit movie *Twister*, which required a great deal of physical endurance.

There are some days when you feel strong enough to push to the max and you do. Then there are some days when your desire is there but the time isn't. Of course there are days when the baby's bad night the night before has you sleep- and energy-deprived. Every day is different and so you can handle every day differently.

If you don't have a chunk of time available to do an entire workout, use the A.M.–P.M. plan: Do half of your exercises in the morning and the other half later in the day.

If you memorize the exercises we've scripted, you can do them individually anytime, anywhere. So, if you're at work and you have a few minutes of downtime, close the door and do some lunges. Do accordions when you're waiting for your hairdresser. Do biceps curls with the baby when you're watching TV.

If you're somewhere where you can take the stairs instead of the elevator, climb stairs. If you have to go to the market, walk, if it's at all possible. Take the baby in her stroller and put the groceries in a basket attached to the stroller. You can then push the baby and the groceries home. The added weight will create resistance and give you a workout.

Whatever you do, don't make excuses for not exercising. Excuses are an exercise in futility. They won't get you anywhere. We will. Follow us.

Postpregnancy Workout—Month 3

Start with our warm-up. It's on page 7. You can do the warm-up

once, twice, or even three times before you start our routine. The better condition you're in, the faster your body warms up. If you want to avoid the risk of injuring your muscles, it's most important never to start cold.

After you've got your heart pumping, take hold of your baby and start exercising.

PROPS

- Chair
- Hand weights
- Rubber exercise band, panty hose, or tights
- Baby

Plié with Baby

We did this move with the baby last month. Now that your baby has gained weight, baby's added size will give you added resistance. And we've increased the number of repetitions on these.

Stand with your legs wider than shoulder-width apart. Your feet are positioned at ten o'clock and two o'clock. Your knees are slightly bent. Baby is cradled in your arms with his or her back parallel to your chest and body in a vertical position.

Bend your knees and lower. Come down to where your butt is

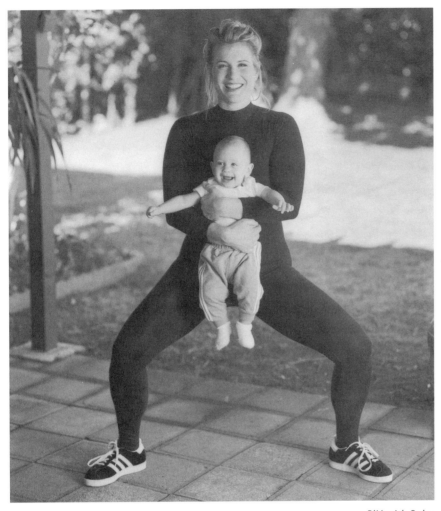

Plié with Baby

about level with your knees and your knees are pointed out over your toes. Make this move straight down. Do not tilt your torso forward. Do not dip lower than your knees.

Now squeeze your gluts as you lift up. Come back up to the starting position with your knees slightly bent. Don't lock your knees straight.

Do 15 of these pliés with your baby.

Note: If you find these pliés too easy, you can do them as pulses.

You're in the same plié position, with your legs wider than shoulder-width apart and your feet positioned at ten o'clock and two o'clock. Your knees are slightly bent, your baby is cradled in your arms. Raise and lower slightly.

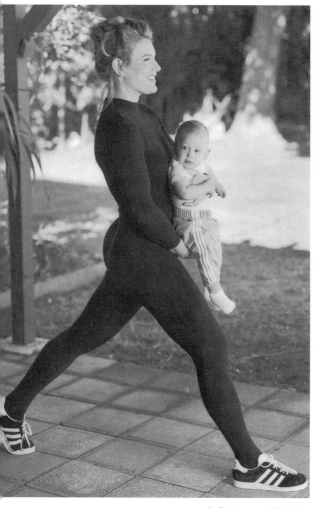
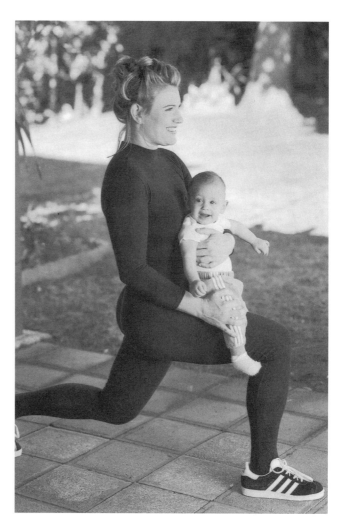

Split Lunge with Baby

Split Lunge with Baby

Cradle the baby against your chest. Alternate legs as you do these split forward lunges.

Stand with your feet shoulder-width apart. Step forward with your right leg, bending your right knee so that your right quad is parallel to the floor. Do not bend your knee further forward than the toes of your right foot. Bend your left knee down toward the floor. Keep your weight on your right foot. Your left quad is facing forward and your left foot is behind you. Keep your upper body straight as you hold the baby.

Now push back to the starting position by pushing up on your right heel.

Alternate legs. Step forward with your left leg. Bend your left knee, making sure your knee is aligned with your ankle. Your right leg is behind you, your knee bending down toward the floor. Keep your weight on your left foot. Keeping your upper body straight, push back through your left heel to the starting position.

Repeat these moves for a total of 20 reps: 10 reps with your right leg forward, alternating with 10 reps with your left leg forward.

You will feel these lunges in your gluts and your quads.

Overhead Press

You're going to need weights for this. If you've been working with 3-pound weights until now, it's time to increase the resistance, so this month you should try 5-pound weights.

Get into your basic standing position with your legs shoulder-width apart and your knees bent slightly. Your arms, holding the weights, are down at your sides.

Standing steady, bring up your arms, bending them with your palms facing forward. Straighten your arms as you lift your hands and weights overhead. Hold your fully extended arms up overhead for a beat, then lower your arms to their bent-at-the-elbow starting position.

You exhale on every lift and inhale on every return.

Do 20 reps of this overhead press.

Reverse Fly

We're going to continue working your shoulders and upper back a

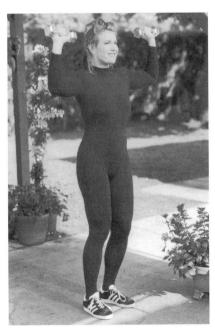

Overhead Press

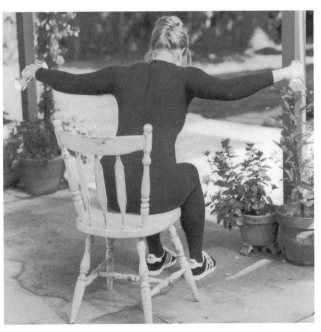

Reverse Fly

little harder this month. We're going back to the reverse fly, which we did in your pregnancy workout. You can use the 3-pound weights you used back then or, if you're feeling strong enough, try this with your 5-pound weights.

Sit squarely on the chair seat. Take one weight in each hand, holding them loosely with your palms facing back. Your knees are bent and your feet are planted together on the floor. Lean forward so that your upper body comes down toward your quads. You can rest lightly on your quads. Keep your back flat at all times. Your face is looking down.

Raise your arms out to your sides. Your elbows are slightly bent as you "fly" your arms back, squeezing your shoulder blades together. Your elbows end up level with your upper back. Now lower your arms back down to your sides and repeat.

Count each lift of the arms up and down as 1 rep. Do 10 reps to complete 1 set. Then repeat a second set of 10.

Triceps Dip

Even if you've lost every ounce of "baby fat," the back of the arm (triceps) is an area where women have a natural tendency to get flabby. This month we're going to help you work that area even harder than before.

Move your butt to the edge of the chair seat. Your legs are bent at the knees and your feet are flat on the floor. Place your hands behind you on the seat with your knuckles facing forward. Bend your elbows as you take your butt off the seat and lower it so that it's level with the edge of the chair, your hands, and your quads.

Dip your butt down toward the floor. The lower you go, the more you'll feel it in the back of your arms, or your triceps. As you get stronger, you'll be able to go lower, but never go lower than is comfortable and don't let your elbows pass your shoulders at the end of the exercise. Your butt should never touch the floor.

Inhale as you lower and exhale as you lift up.

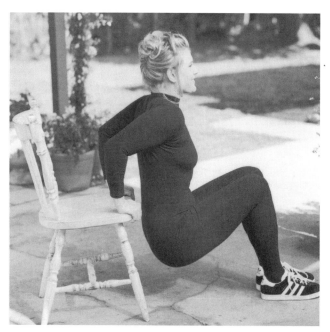

Triceps Dip

Do 15 of these triceps dips.

We're going to do the remainder of this workout on the floor. If you do wind up dividing your workout during the day, the following is a good group of seven exercises to do together since they're all done on the floor.

Side Leg Lift with Weight

We'll start with the side leg lifts and this time we suggest you use a weight for these.

Get onto your right side with your right arm extended in line with your body. Rest your head on this arm. Bend your knees and bring them up toward your chest.

They should be at an angle to your hips that's between 45 and 90 degrees.

Your hips and legs are stacked and you place your weight on your working leg, the left one. Using your left hand, hold the weight in place just below your hip on your left outer thigh. Lift your left leg so that your knee comes up a little higher than your hip. You should not roll backward. If you do, you've lifted too high.

Squeeze your gluts as you lower your leg. Do not rest your working leg. Lift it again. The hand weight is giving you resistance so that your outer thigh muscle works harder.

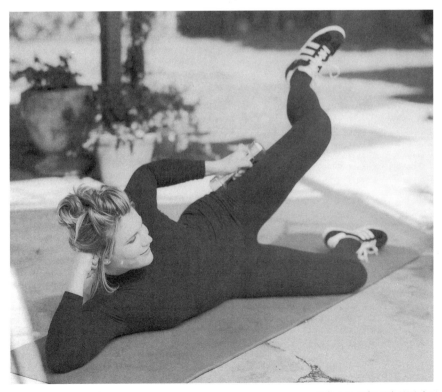

Side Leg Lift with Weight

Do 20 reps, then switch sides.
Get down on your left side and rest your head on your left extended arm. Bend your knees and place the weight on your right outer thigh, holding it in place with your right hand. Now lift your right leg up so that it comes higher than your right hip. Be careful not to roll backward. Lower your leg—don't rest it—then lift again.

Do 20 reps.

Straight-Leg Lift

Let's keep working that hip and outer thigh area (gluteus medius). Stay on the floor, switch back onto your right side, and straighten your legs. They remain stacked so that the inside of your left knee rests on the inside of your right knee. Keep your lower leg slightly bent for balance. Your left hand is in front of your chest, anchoring you in place.

Squeeze your butt and tilt your pelvis up slightly. Now lift your left leg, keeping your knee

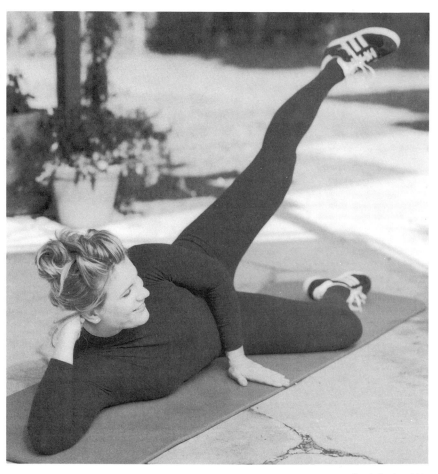

Straight-Leg Lift

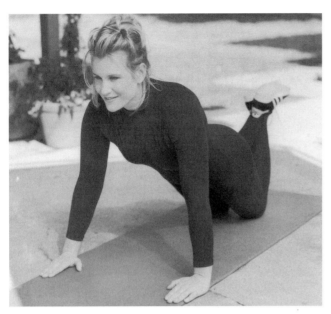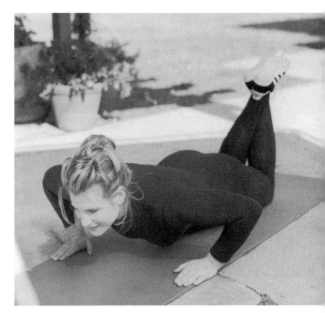

Push-Up

facing forward. Don't roll forward or backward when you lift. Your leg will not even lift hip high if you're squeezing hard. Lower your leg. Don't rest it. Lift again. Do 20 reps. Switch sides.

Lie on your left side and extend your legs straight. Place your right arm in front of your chest for support. Squeeze your gluts and tilt your pelvis up slightly. Don't tilt as you lift your straightened right leg almost hip high. Lower your leg. Do 20 reps with your right leg.

Push-Up

Push-ups are probably the singularly most effective exercise for working your total upper body: triceps, pectorals, and anterior deltoids.

Come onto your hands and knees. Cross your feet at the ankles. Your hands are parallel with your shoulders, placed a little wider than your chest. Your fingers are pointing forward and your head is forward with your face looking down toward the floor.

Exhale as you push up. Tighten your abs and squeeze your gluts at the same time, which gives support to your lower back. Your back should remain straight; be careful not to let it sag. Inhale and lower toward the floor but do not rest on the floor; push up again. When you get to the top, straighten your arms but do not lock your elbows.

Count each push-up and lower as 1 rep. Do 8 reps, rest a beat, and then do 8 more push-ups.

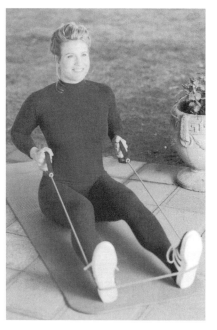

Seated Row

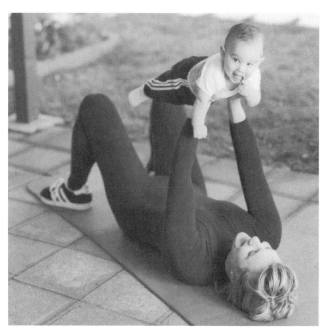

Chest Press with Baby

Seated Row

Turn around and sit on the floor. Take your rubber stretch band, a pair of old panty hose, or tights. Extend your legs in front of you and keep your knees slightly bent. Hold the ends of the band or hose in your hands and run it under your feet, bringing the ends up toward your waist. Your palms are facing inward.

The band should be secure in your hands as you pull back on it. Your elbows will bend back as you pull as far as you can, squeezing your shoulder blades together. You'll feel the work in your biceps and rear deltoids.

Count each pull back as 1 rep. Do 20 reps.

Chest Press with Baby

If the baby is nearby, it would be nice to include him or her in this chest press. The lifting motion generally puts a smile on baby's face. We know the results of these chest presses will put a smile on your face.

Lie down while you're holding the baby under his or her arms, perpendicular to you and facing you. Bend your knees slightly and sit the baby on your abs. Lift the baby up without lifting your head, neck, or shoulders off the floor. Hold the baby up for a beat and then lower baby back onto your abs. Count each lift, hold, and lower as 1 rep. Do 8 reps. Rest a beat and then do another 8 reps.

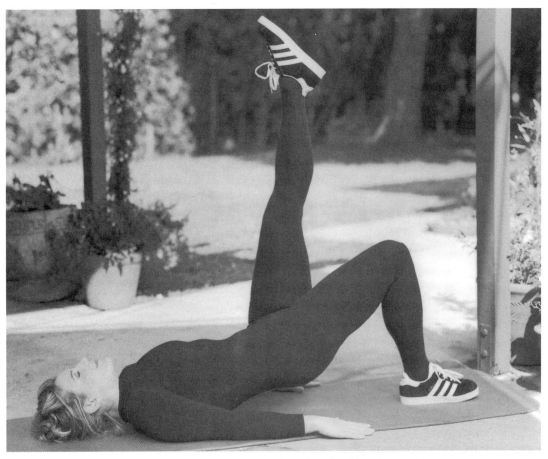

Pelvic Tilt with Bridge, One Leg Up

Pelvic Tilt with Bridge, One Leg Up

We're going to change the action on this a little. You can keep the baby with you or you can do these while the baby watches.

First, without the baby: You're on your back and your knees are bent. Now lift your left leg so that it is extended straight up. This will put all your weight onto your right leg as you push up from your right heel. Tilt your pelvis up so

that your butt squeezes up off the floor. Your abs tighten as you exhale. Your lower back comes slightly up off the floor. Hold for a beat and lower. Do 15 reps with your left leg extended.

Remain on your back with your knees bent. This time lift up your right leg so that it is extended straight up. This will put all your weight onto your left leg as you push up from your left heel. Tilt your pelvis up so that your gluts squeeze up off the floor.

Your abs tighten as you exhale. Your lower back comes slightly up off the floor. Hold for a beat and lower. Do 15 of these bridges with your right leg extended.

Now, with the baby: Rest baby against your left quad while she or he sits on your abs. Her or his weight will add more resistance, making your left leg work harder.

Count each pelvic tilt and lower as 1 rep. Do 15 reps with your right leg up and extended. Switch working legs.

Keep your right foot on the floor, with your right knee bent.

The baby rests on your right quad as you extend your left leg straight up into the air. Now tilt your pelvis up. Squeeze your butt and lower back off the floor. Hold for a beat and lower. Do 15 reps with your left leg up and extended.

Crunch with Pelvic Tilt

You can keep the baby resting on your abs if you'd like or you can ask baby to watch you crunch on your own.

You're still on your back. Clasp your hands behind your head for support. Bend your knees, keeping your feet flat on

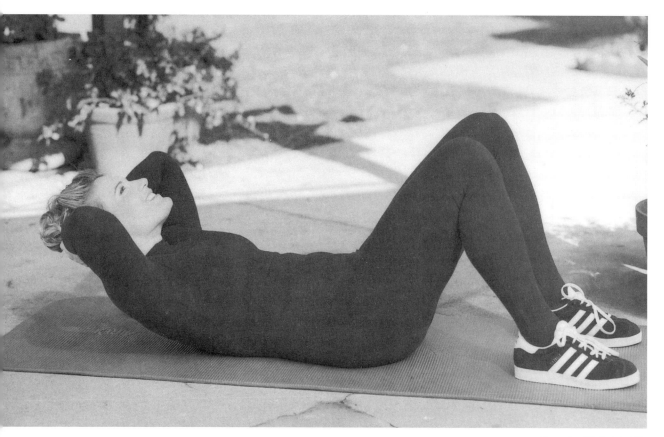

Crunch with Pelvic Tilt

the floor. Tilt your pelvis as you lift your head and shoulders off the floor toward your bent knees. Imagine your bottom rib and your hip bones coming closer together as you make this move. Squeeze your PC muscle with every crunch. Lower your shoulders but don't rest at the bottom. Crunch up again.

Do 20 reps. Rest a beat and then do 20 more.

Now do the cool-down (see page 16).

You've just completed your third month postpartum exercise program. You can repeat this performance throughout the month as it is scripted or you can add more repetitions. If you prefer, you can go back to any earlier workouts and borrow moves from them. The idea is to challenge yourself and to keep yourself motivated.

Again, don't worry if you don't have a chunk of time that will allow you to do all the exercises. Do what you can when you can. And remember, always listen to your body. It will let you know what's best for you.

Keep up the good work.

POSTPREGNANCY WORKOUT
MONTH 3 SUMMARY*

EXERCISE	REPS	SETS
Plié with Baby	15	1
Split Lunge with Baby		
right	10	1
left	10	1
Overhead Press	20	1
Reverse Fly	10	2
Triceps Dip	15	1
Side Leg Lift with Weight		
right	20	1
left	20	1
Straight-Leg Lift		
right	20	1
left	20	1
Push-Up	8	2
Seated Row	20	1
Chest Press with Baby	8	2
Pelvic Tilt with Bridge, One Leg Up		
right	15	1
left	15	1
Crunch with Pelvic Tilt	20	2

* Repeat exercises or add sets at your discretion.

six

Striking Distance

Month 4: Getting Back to Where You Once Belonged

By now, life with baby has settled into more of a routine. You may be back at work, your stamina has increased, and, with the working out you've been doing, your body is, we hope, starting to look like it used to.

Each one of our "Primetime Moms" found that, because she had worked out prior to her pregnancy and during her pregnancy, her postpregnancy shape-up routine helped her regain control over her body. But not everyone is as lucky as Michelle, who was pretty much back to normal within the first few months. It took Sheryl Lowe ten months to get her shape back after gaining 38 pounds with her first son. Harriet Posner, whose legal practice keeps her in the office a minimum of ten hours a day, finally got back her pre-pregnancy figure about 18 months after she gave birth to her second son (she gained 28 pounds with that pregnancy). Jami reached her weight goal in eight months, and Rita took off that extra weight she gained during breast-feeding within four months. By the time Meg was four months postpregnancy, she was in such good shape that she could take off to shoot *Sleepless in Seattle*.

Each Primetime Mom had different workout schedules. For instance, Michelle kept up her five-day-a-week workout, while Sheryl worked out with Kathy four days a week for the ten months it took her to get back into shape. Harriet worked with Kathy two days a week and played tennis twice every weekend for three hours each time. And Jami worked out three times a week.

As for Kathy, by the time she reached her fourth postpregnancy month, she was back in her old jeans, but she hadn't lost even one ounce between two-and-a-half months and four months postpregnancy. And for Kathy that was frustrating.

Her workout schedule varied from day to day during the first few months after her twins were born. Some weeks she worked out every day; sometimes she worked out a couple of hours during the day. Other weeks, she was so busy doing photo shoots, taking business meetings, filming an infomercial for her new Workout Ball, and flying to New York to appear on the *Today* show that she barely had time to do even one leg lift.

Yet, somehow, when she did steal an hour at 5:30 A.M. (working out with Michelle), she found herself feeling better and more energetic throughout the rest of her long day. She also took time to adjust her mind to the fact that her body was going to shape up at its own pace and that no matter how many hours she worked out in a day, a week, or throughout those first months, her scale was not going to be the measure of her progress—her attitude would be.

And so it should be with you. We've got the script for you to follow. We've even made it more challenging and more interesting. You can follow it exactly as it's written or you can do your own interpretations. Do extra repetitions, split the moves up between the day or night, add on a couple of last month's exercises, increase your weights, or change your aerobics workout (you should be able to go as long as 45 to 60 minutes). Walk at lunchtime, do some of this month's exercises on Monday night, and do the rest on Tuesday night. Be creative but be creative four to six times a week if you want quicker results. Just remember, it's all in the attitude!

Postpregnancy Workout—Month 4

Turn to our warm-up on page 7. Please use this warm-up, or do some form of aerobics, before you start your workout.

- Chair
- Hand weights
- Baby

Plié with Baby

Baby's putting on weight and he or she can help you take off weight again this month.

Cradle baby in your arms so that his or her head rests on one of your arms and his or her lower body is supported with your other arm.

Stand with your legs more than shoulder-width apart. Your toes should be pointed and at 10 o'clock and 2 o'clock on the face of your imaginary clock.

Keeping your upper body straight, lower your body by bending your knees in the direction of your toes. Bring your body down so that your butt is almost at a 45-degree angle to your knees, and your knees are at a 45-degree angle to your ankles. Make sure your knees do not go beyond your toes or you will place too much pressure on your knees.

Lift up slowly, squeezing your butt as you lift. Come up to where your knees remain soft or slightly bent.

Count each plié and lift as 1 rep. Do 10 reps.

Pulse with Baby

You're going to add another move here: a pulse. A pulse is a slight lift and slight lowering of your torso. Count each lift and lower as 1 rep.

Continue with another plié but when you get to the bottom, do 10 pulses. Return to doing 1 set of 10 slow pliés.

SUPERSET 1

Overhead Press and Reverse Fly

Overhead Press

We've lowered the repetitions on this move because we're giving you a superset to do here. A *superset* is a group of two or more exercises that work opposing muscle groups without a break between the exercises. Try to use 5-pound weights if you've been using 3 pounds until now.

Stand in the basic position with one weight in each hand. Keep your pelvis neutral while you bend your arms up with your palms forward. Straighten your arms as you lift them until they're fully extended over your head, exhaling as you lift. Press up and hold for a beat, then return your arms to their original bent-at-the-elbow position.

Do 12 reps and go right to the next exercise.

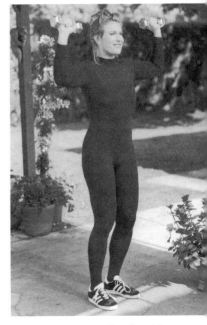

Overhead Press

Reverse Fly

Take your chair and weights and sit on the edge of the chair. Bend forward at the waist. Your arms start down at your sides. Your head is straight—as if it were an extension of the top of your spine. Your head is facing down and your eyes focus on your toes.

Lift your arms out to the sides and up to shoulder level as you exhale. Keep your elbows slightly bent as you squeeze your shoulder blades together. Your palms are facing the floor. You'll feel the back of your shoulders and your upper arms working. Return your arms down so that your palms and weights are facing your feet.

Do 12 of these reverse flys.

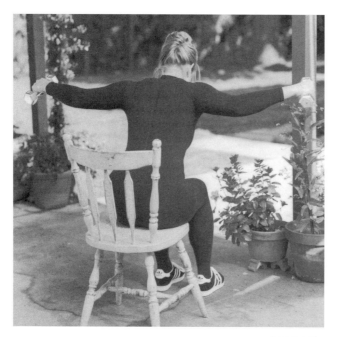

Reverse Fly

Triceps Kick-Back

Use your 3-pound weights for this unless you're very strong, then you can use the 5-pound weights; or if you want to, you can alternate between the 3- and 5-pound weights between sets.

We'll start with your right arm. With the chair on your left, stand on your right leg, keeping that knee soft, and place your left knee on your chair. Extend your upper body across the seat of your chair, supporting your body with your left hand on the chair seat. Balance your body so your back is flat and steady. Bring your right

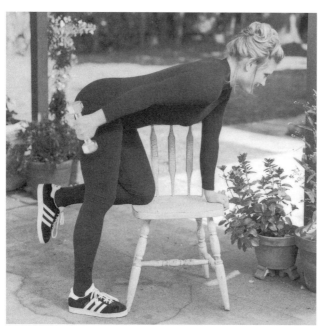

Triceps Kick-Back

arm up so your upper arm is parallel to your back.

With your right palm facing in toward your body, exhale and extend your forearm back, keeping your elbow in a straight line with your shoulder. This exercise will work best if only your forearm moves and not your elbow. Squeeze your triceps on the extension and inhale as you return down to the starting position. Do 25 reps of these kick-backs with your right arm. Turn and switch sides.

Stand on your left leg, keeping a slight bend in the knee and rest your right knee on the chair. Bend from the waist so that your upper body is across the chair seat. Support your upper body with your right arm on the chair seat. Bend your left elbow so that your upper arm is parallel to your back. Your palm and weight are facing in toward your body.

Exhale and extend your left arm back so that it is straight and parallel to the floor. Do not move your elbow. Squeeze the triceps and inhale as you bring your forearm back down to its original position.

Do 25 reps of these kick-backs to complete 1 set. Do 1 more set of 25 kick-backs with each arm.

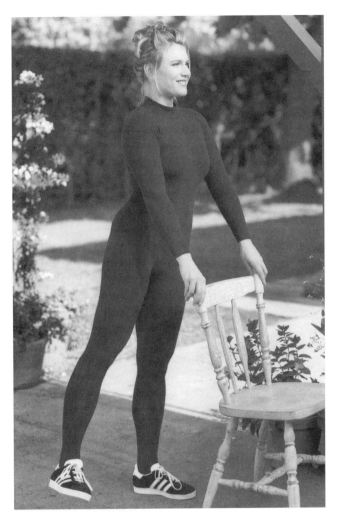

Standing Straight-Leg Lift

Standing Straight-Leg Lift

Stand behind your chair at arm's length, facing the back of your chair. Lightly hold on to the chair back for support. Your legs are about shoulder-width apart and your knees are bent slightly. Tilt your pelvis up.

Now with your right foot facing forward, lift your straightened right leg out from the center of your body. You will not be able to lift it very high when you keep your hips in the forward position. Lower your leg so that your foot grazes the floor and lift it out to the right side again. Do 20 reps of this standing straight-leg lift then switch working legs.

Your right leg is now your supporting leg and, with your left foot facing forward, lift your left leg out to the side. Remember to keep your pelvis tilted up. Lower your left leg and repeat. Do 20 reps of this standing straight-leg lift to complete 1 set.

Do a second set of 20 reps with each leg.

SUPERSET 2

One-Arm Row and Push-Up

One-Arm Row

Go around to the front of the chair with one of your 5-pound weights, and again put your left knee on the chair seat. Bend from the waist so that your torso is across the chair seat. Your left arm supports your torso.

Now, starting with your right arm down at your side, palm and weight facing inward, lift your weight up by bending your elbow and bringing it up so that it comes just past your shoulder. Lower your hand and weight back down toward the floor. Do 15 of these rows with your right arm, then switch working arms.

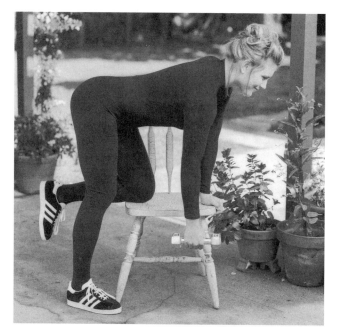

One-Arm Row

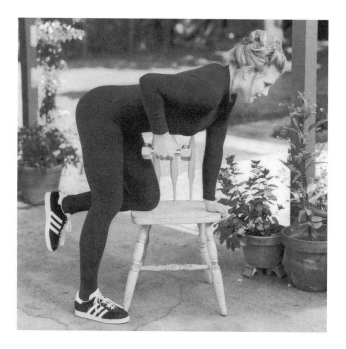

Place your right knee on the chair seat, bend your upper body from the waist, and support your upper body with your right arm. Your left arm is down at your side and, while keeping your upper body straight, bring your hand and weight up by bending your elbow. Your elbow should come just past your shoulder. Then lower your hand and weight back down toward the floor. Do 15 of these rows with your left arm to complete 1 set. Do a second set of 15 reps with each arm.

Move right on to the second exercise in the superset.

Push-Up

Get on your hands and knees on the floor. Cross your feet at the ankles. Your hands are parallel with your shoulders, your fingers point forward, and your head is forward, face down.

Exhale as you push up and simultaneously tighten your abs and squeeze your gluts. Your back must remain straight—beware of the tendency to let your back sag. Now inhale and lower toward the floor but do not rest on the floor; push up again. When you get to the top, straighten your arms but do not lock your elbows. Keep them flexible to help you get back

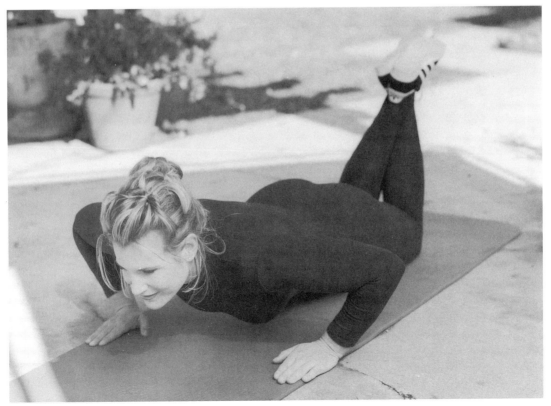

Push-Up

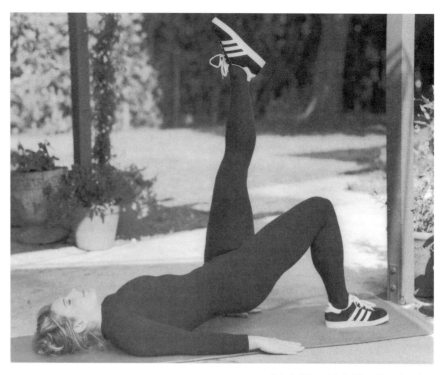

Pelvic Tilt with Bridge, One Leg Up

down. Do 12 push-ups to complete 1 set. Rest a beat and repeat a second set of 12 reps.

Pelvic Tilt with Bridge

Get onto your back and bend your knees. Your feet are flat on the floor and your hands are resting at your sides. Your head, neck, and shoulders are still throughout this entire exercise.

Tilt your pelvis up and squeeze your gluts up. Both your gluts and your lower back come up off the floor as you exhale, pulling in on your abs. Slowly lower your back and gluts onto the floor and then repeat the pelvic tilt. You can squeeze your PC muscle with every tilt. Do 20 reps of these pelvic tilts with bridge.

Pelvic Tilt with Bridge, One Leg Up

Remain on your back with your knees bent. This time lift up your right leg so that it is extended straight up. This will put all your weight onto your left leg as you push up from your left heel. Tilt your pelvis up so that your gluts squeeze up off the floor. Your abs tighten as you exhale. Your lower back comes slightly up off the floor. Hold for a beat and lower. Do 15 of these bridges with your right leg extended then switch legs.

Lift your left leg so it is extended straight up. Your weight will now be on your right leg as you push up from your right heel. Tilt your pelvis up so that your gluts squeeze up off the floor. As you exhale, your abs tighten. Your lower back comes slightly up off the floor and you hold for a beat and lower. Do 15 of these bridges with your left leg extended.

SUPERSET 3

Crunch—with Pelvic Tilt, with Knees Up, with Straight Legs Up— and Reverse Curl

Crunch

Lie on your back with your feet hip-width apart and your knees bent. Your feet are flat on the floor and your hands are clasped behind your head. Keep your chin off your chest as you exhale and pull your abs in toward your spine while you lift your head, neck, and shoulders off the floor. Do not pull on your head or neck with your hands. Lower your head and shoulders back down onto the floor. Do 20 reps of these crunches.

Crunch with Pelvic Tilt

Stay right where you are in the same position: knees bent, feet flat on the floor, hands behind your head. This time tilt your pelvis as you lift your upper body toward your bent knees. Imagine your bottom rib and your pelvis coming closer together as you move. Lower your shoulders but don't rest. Do 20 reps.

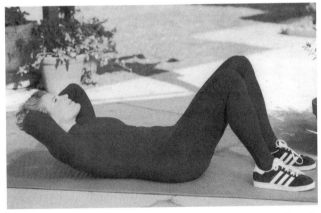

Crunch

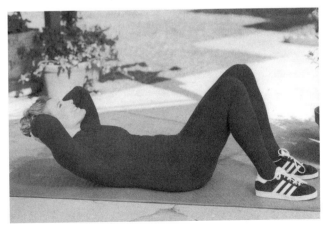

Crunch with Pelvic Tilt

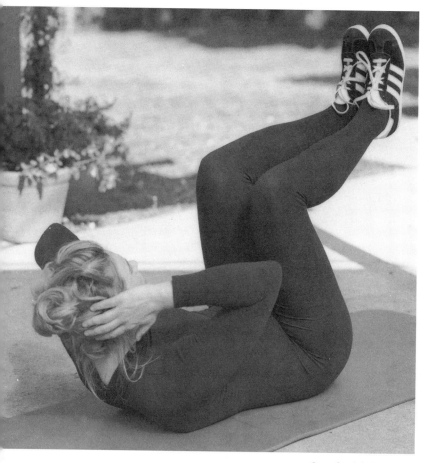

Crunch with Knees Up

Crunch with Knees Up

This time you're going to lift your knees so your legs form a right angle to your hips. Your hands are still behind your head. Lift your torso up toward your bent knees. Exhale as you lift and inhale as you lower, but do not touch the floor with your shoulders.

Do 20 reps.

Crunch with Straight Legs Up

Straighten your legs up from their bent-knee position. Lift your hips and legs as you lift your head and shoulders up toward your straight legs. As you lower your upper body, bring your hips back down onto the floor. Do 20 reps.

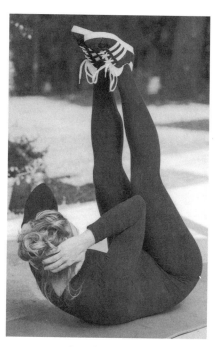

Crunch with Straight Legs Up

Reverse Curl

Keep your legs lifted. This time your upper body stays flat on the floor as you lift your hips and legs up off the floor. Then lower your hips down and up again. Remember, you do not move your head or shoulders. You want to isolate the lower part of your abs with this work. Do 20 reps.

Take a deep breath and move on to the cool-down, which is on page 16.

You did it! We know that wasn't easy, but it wasn't supposed to be. This month's workout is a challenge, but as you meet this challenge, you'll feel better about yourself. And you should start noticing some results. Even if your scale is stuck, like Kathy's has been, your strength is growing and your attitude is making you feel better no matter how much you weigh. The trick is to give yourself a chance to be the best that you can be. Keep working at it.

Next month is a superset month. You'll need to be ready for it so try and do the exercises you did today as many as six times a week. You'll be surprised at how effective this kind of schedule can be.

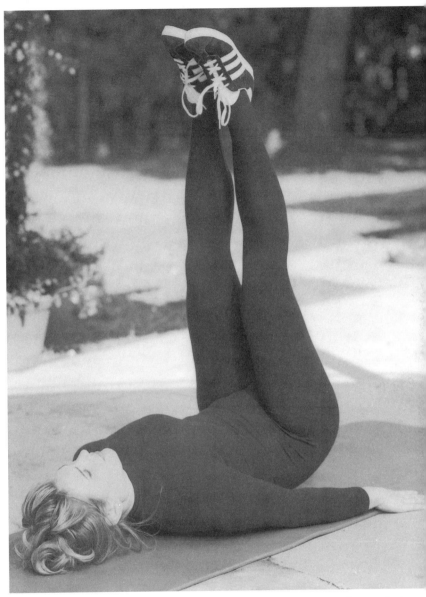

Reverse Curl

POSTPREGNANCY WORKOUT
MONTH 4 SUMMARY*

EXERCISE	REPS	SETS
Plié with Baby	10	1
Pulse with Baby	10	1

SUPERSET 1

Overhead Press	12	1
Reverse Fly	12	1

Triceps Kick-Back

right	25	2
left	25	2

Standing Straight-Leg Lift

right	20	2
left	20	2

SUPERSET 2

One-Arm Row

right	15	2
left	15	2

Push-Up	12	2

* Repeat exercises or add sets at your discretion.

EXERCISE	REPS	SETS
Pelvic Tilt with Bridge	20	1
Pelvic Tilt with Bridge, One Leg Up		
right	15	1
left	15	1

Crunch	20	1
Crunch with Pelvic Tilt	20	1
Crunch with Knees Up	20	1
Crunch with Straight Legs Up	20	1
Reverse Curl	20	1

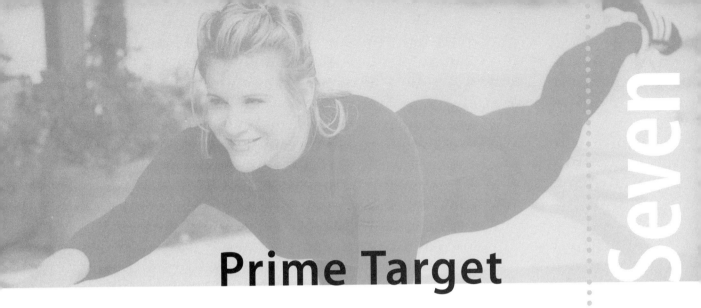

Seven

Prime Target

Month 5: Target Your Prime-time Postpregnancy Figure

his month your baby's weight is up to an average of 16 to 18 pounds. With all your workouts, yours should be down at least that much, if not as much as 20 pounds or more. As we've been telling you, the best way to hit your target weight is with a good cardio workout that you do faithfully. By this month you should be able to do a 40- to 60-minute cardiovascular workout four to six times a week. And, if you add on our 20-minute workout, you're talking about a serious dedication of time.

We know that with a new baby, a career, and a mate all needing your attention you might be finding it difficult to find that time. Unless you can afford to hire lots of help, you've got to be creative in finding ways to create time for your workouts and you've got to be creative about including your baby in your workout plans.

One Saturday night after Cooper and Payton were born, Kathy's father-in-law offered to baby-sit the babies so Kathy and her husband, Billy, could go out to a movie. Kathy took her father-in-law up on his offer to baby-sit, but she and Billy got only as far as their exercise equipment. It meant more to Kathy to have some quiet time to work out than to sit in a movie theater.

If you set your mind to thinking in that direction you, too, can find ways to bring your exercise time into being. If you have family close by, ask your mother or sister to watch the baby while you work out in another room of the house. If you don't have family, you can hire a baby-sitter for an hour or two, or look for a fitness center that provides day care.

Work out during baby's nap time. That's what Rita Wilson Hanks and Sheryl Lowe did. Or if Rob Lowe was home from work Sheryl asked him to watch the baby while she exercised. Harriet Posner made a deal with her husband. She got Thursday nights and Saturday mornings off from the kids in exchange for two days that he got off. Harriet used those times to work out with Kathy.

You can find new ways to adapt your workout to baby. Look in magazines for advertised products that will accommodate the baby in your workout. There are baby joggers, strollers, and Snuglis that you can use to include your baby. Rita kept her baby in a Snugli on her back when she did step aerobics. The baby loved it and Rita had fun working out with him until he got too heavy for comfort.

When Cooper got fussy, Kathy cradled him in her arms while she worked out on the exercise bike. The steady motion calmed him and Kathy got an extra aerobics session in for herself.

It's important for you to be inventive, too. You can't look like Michelle, Meg, Rita, Jami, or Kathy without trying. *They* can't look like they do without trying. Getting into shape means letting nothing get in your way.

This month, we're going to step up your workouts with supersets. All the combinations of exercises we have scripted for you are designed to maximize your efforts. Our supersets mean super shape and strength for your body's prime target areas. Even if your weight hasn't been dropping as quickly as you'd like, these moves will sculpt your muscles so that as the weight does come off, you'll look shapelier and healthier.

We do not call for you to use your baby this month. We feel that with supersets we don't want you to take the time between moves to take care of baby. If you want to work out with your baby, by all means hold on to him or her during leg lunges, pliés, and bridges.

We are giving you six supersets this month. You can divide them up and do them throughout the day or you can work the A.M.–P.M. plan, half of them in the morning and half in the evening. We don't think you should divide up the supersets themselves. So, for instance, if you want to do three supersets in the morning and three in the afternoon, great, but once you start a superset, follow through with it. It's designed to maximize results and the results will be worth it.

As we've said before, you can combine any of the exercises in this month's workout with exercises from past months. You can target a trouble spot like your abs and increase the number of repetitions you do in the abs work, or you can increase the weight of your hand weights for your upper-body work.

Postpregnancy Workout—Month 5

Even if you've done a 60-minute aerobic session, turn to our warm-up on page 7. It will better prepare your body and your mind for our superset month.

PROPS

• Chair
• Hand weights
• Rubber exercise band or panty hose

turn to our warm-up on page 7.

SUPERSET 1

Lunge and Plié

Alternating Leg Lunge

We'll try this alternating leg lunge without a chair this month. Stand with your feet hip-width apart. Your hands are on your hips and your upper body is straight. Step your right leg forward one big step, bend both knees, and lower your body. Keep your weight distributed evenly on both feet. The heel of your left foot is raised off the floor. Make sure your front knee is over your ankle. Now push back into the starting position.

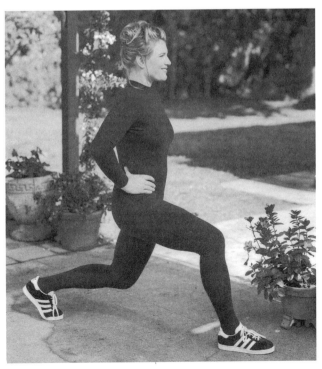

Alternating Leg Lunge

Alternate legs. Step your left leg forward one big step, bend both knees and lower your body. Your right heel is raised off the floor. Keep your weight evenly distributed on both feet. Your front knee is over your ankle. Now push back to starting position.

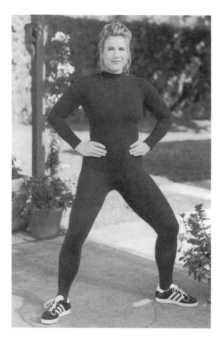

Plié

Plié

Shift your feet into the plié position. Your feet are more than shoulder-width apart and they are pointed in the ten o'clock and two o'clock directions. Your knees are slightly bent.

Your hands are still on your hips and your upper body is straight as you bend your knees

out over your toes. Lower your butt so it's even with your knees—but no lower. Now squeeze your gluts as you slowly lift up to the starting position and then lower and lift again.

The alternating leg lunge and two pliés equal 1 superset. The rhythm is: lunge right leg, lunge left leg, plié down twice, and repeat.

Do 10 of these supersets.

SUPERSET 2

Triceps Kick-Back, Overhead Press, Biceps Curl, and Seated Row

Get your chair, hand weights, and band. We hope you're using 5-pound weights by now.

Triceps Kick-Back

We'll start with your right arm. Stand on your right leg and place your left knee on your chair. Your torso is extended forward above and across the seat of your chair. Balance your body so your back is flat and steady. Bring your right arm up so your upper arm is parallel to your back. Keep your left knee relaxed to make sure your back is flat.

With your right palm and weight facing inward, extend your

arm back, keeping the elbow in a straight line with your shoulder. Exhale and squeeze your triceps, then inhale as you return down to the starting position.

Do 15 reps, then switch working arms.

Your right knee comes up onto the chair and your torso is extended forward so it's above and across the seat of your chair. Your left leg is standing and your knee is slightly bent. Bring your left arm up so your upper arm is parallel to your back. With your left palm and weight facing inward, extend your arm back, making sure your left elbow stays in a straight line with your shoulder. Exhale and squeeze your triceps, not your hand weight. Inhale as you return to the starting position.

Do 15 reps with your left arm. Come off the chair and pick up your second hand weight.

Overhead Press

Stand in the basic position of feet shoulder-width apart. Bend your arms up with your palms and weights facing forward. Straighten your arms as you lift them until they're fully extended over your head, exhaling as you go. Press up and hold for a beat, then return your arms to their original bent-at-the-elbow position. Do 15 reps of the overhead press.

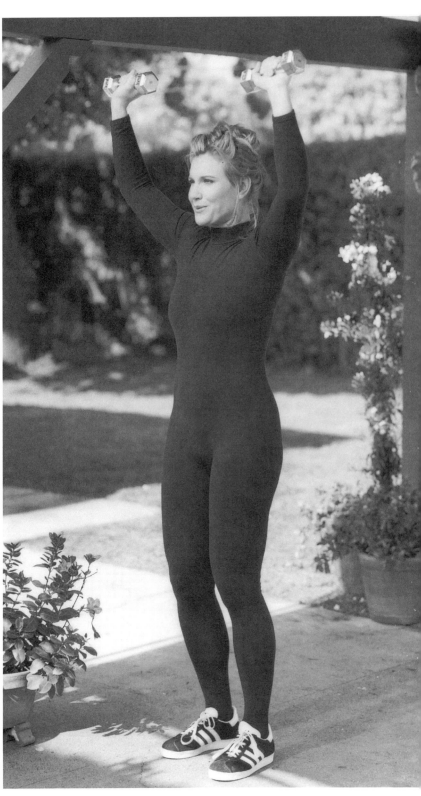

Overhead Press

Biceps Curl

Bring your arms down so they are bent and at your sides. Press your elbows into your waist and turn your palms and weights up. Curl your arms up, bringing your weights up toward your shoulders. Squeeze your biceps as you curl up and when you return your arms to the starting position. Exhale as you curl up and inhale as your arms come down to waist level.

Do 20 reps of these biceps curls. Get down on the floor with your rubber exercise band or your panty hose.

Seated Row

Sit on the floor with your legs extended in front of you but do not straighten them. Keep your knees slightly bent. If you're using an old pair of panty hose or tights, hold the waistband in one hand and the two feet of the hose together in the other hand.

Run the band or hose under your flexed feet. Your hands are facing inward as you pull back on the band. Your elbows bend back as you pull. Pull as far back as you can, feeling the work in your biceps and rear deltoids. Release slowly and bring your arms into their original straight position.

Do 15 reps of these seated rows.

Seated Row

Pelvic Tilt with Bridges—Pulse, Weight on Heels, Right Leg Up/Kegel, Left Leg Up/Kegel—and Pelvic Tilt Without Bridge

Pelvic Tilt with Bridge

Go down onto the floor and lay flat on your back. Keep your hands resting at your sides and bend your knees. Your feet are slightly apart and flat on the floor. Lift your gluts by tilting your pelvis up and squeezing your gluts off the floor. As you lift a little higher, your lower back comes off the floor. Your head, neck, and shoulders are resting comfortably on the floor. Now lower your lower back and gluts and then lift again.

Do 10 reps of this pelvic tilt with bridge.

Pulse

Now squeeze up again and this time pulse at the top. You do this by lifting and lowering slightly.

Do 10 pulses at the top then come back to starting position on the floor.

Weight on Heels

Do not change positions. Lift up the toes on both your feet. Although this is a minor adjustment, it will put more weight onto your heels and so will work your hamstrings harder. Do the same lift up of your butt and lower back off the floor. Squeeze your gluts when you lift.

Do 10 reps of this lifting and lowering of your gluts and lower back. Then lift again but this time pulse at the top. Do 10 reps of this slight lift and lower pulse with your toes up.

Right Leg Up/Kegel

Lower your gluts and bring your feet together. Now lift up your right leg so that it is fully extended. Tilt your pelvis up, pushing up on your left foot so that you work your left glut harder. At the top, when you're squeezing your butt and your lower back is off the floor, squeeze your PC muscle (do a kegel). Then release your PC muscle and lower your gluts and lower back to the floor.

Do 10 of these bridges then switch legs.

Left Leg Up/Kegel

Bring your left leg up and tilt your gluts and lower back off the floor by pressing on your right foot. At

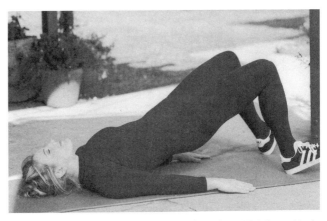

Pelvic Tilt with Bridge—Weight on Heels

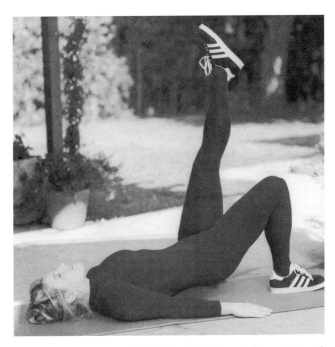

Pelvic Tilt with Bridge—Left Leg Up/Kegel

the top of your lift, do a kegel and release back down to the floor.

Do 10 of these bridges with your left leg extended up.

Pelvic Tilt

Lower your left foot back onto the floor and do pelvic tilts by tilting

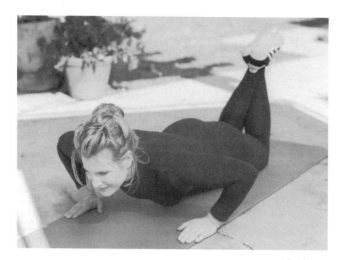

Push-Up

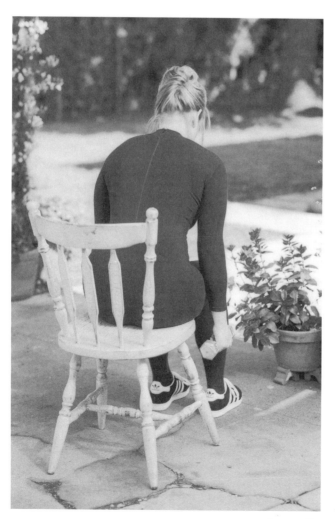

Reverse Fly

your pelvis up and squeezing just your butt off the floor.

Do 10 reps of these pelvic tilts.

Push-Up and Reverse Fly

Push-Up

Still on the floor, get on your hands and knees with your arms straight, your knees bent, and your feet up. Cross your feet at the ankles. Your hands, flat on the floor, are lined up with your shoulders.

Exhale as you push up with your arms. Tighten your abs and your butt as you lift. Make sure you don't arch your back or let it sag. It should remain straight. Your head is forward, extended from your spine—not lifted or dropped.

Inhale as you lower your upper body but do not rest on the floor.

Do 15 of these push-ups.

Now push yourself up onto the chair.

Reverse Fly

Sit at the edge of your chair and bend forward at the waist. Your arms are down at your sides and your palms and weights are facing in. Now exhale and lift your arms out to the sides and up to shoulder level. Make sure you keep your elbows slightly bent as you squeeze your shoulder blades together, working the back of your shoulders.

Return your arms to their starting position as you inhale. Then lift again.

Do 12 of these reverse flys and go back to the floor.

SUPERSET 5

Side Straight-Leg Lift, Arm-Leg Opposition Stretch, and Cat Stretch

Side Straight-Leg Lift

Lie on your left side with your hips and legs stacked. Your left knee is slightly bent while your right leg is straight. The inside of your right knee is facing the inside of your left knee. Your left arm is extended out and your head is resting on your arm. Your right hand is holding a 5-pound weight against the outside of your right thigh.

Flex your right foot and raise your right leg without moving your upper body. Your leg cannot go higher than your hip if your knee is facing straight forward. The lift will leave about two to four inches between your knees. Lower your

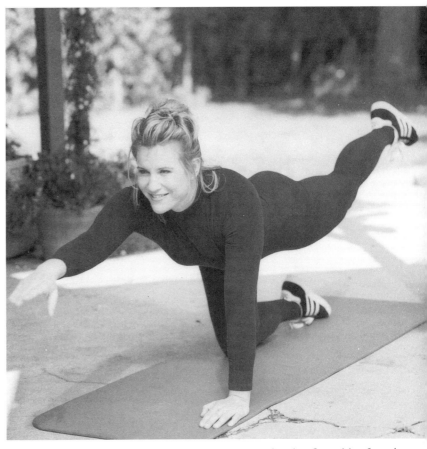

Arm-Leg Opposition Stretch

leg. Don't rest it; instead lift it again.

Do 20 reps with your right leg and then come up on your hands and knees for two stretches.

Arm-Leg Opposition Stretch

You're on your knees and your arms are straight and perpendicular to the floor. Lift your right arm and your left leg off the floor, extending your right arm forward and your left leg back. They are now parallel to the floor.

Balance your torso with your left arm and right knee. Keep your back straight—don't let it arch or slump. Your head is straight, extended from your spine and your eyes are focused on the floor. Stretch your arm and leg and hold this position for a count of 20. Release and come back onto all fours. You're going to switch your working arm and leg.

This time you extend your left arm and your right leg off the floor so that they are parallel to the floor. Your head is extended straight, eyes down. Your back is straight. Support your weight on your right arm and left knee while you stretch your outstretched arm and leg. Hold for a count of 20.

Now repeat these opposition stretches. Start again by extending your right arm and left leg and hold for a count of 20. Switch to extending your left arm and right leg and hold for a count of 20.

Come back on all fours and get ready to do the next stretch.

Cat Stretch

You're still on your hands and knees, your arms are straight, palms flat on the floor, and fingers facing forward.

Round your back up. Concentrate on pulling your abs in toward your spine. Tuck your chin into your chest. Do not lift your hands off the floor as you pull up against gravity. Exhale and release your back and chin. Repeat this cat stretch 4 times. Now lie down on your right side for another set of side leg lifts.

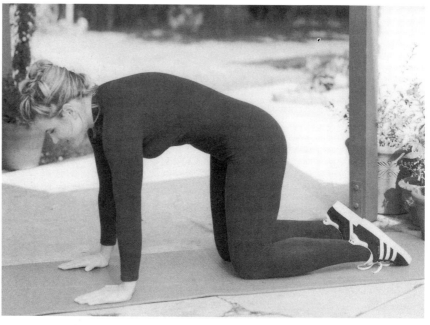

Cat Stretch

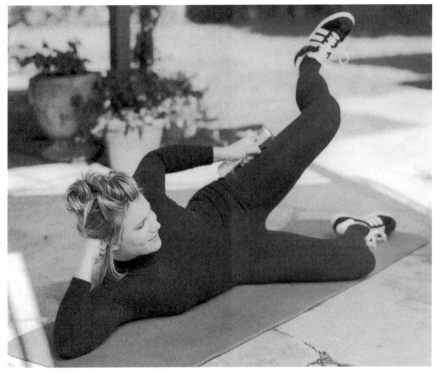

Side Straight-Leg Lift

Side Straight-Leg Lift

You're on your right side, right arm extended on the floor, and your head is resting comfortably on your hand. Your hips are stacked and the inside of your left knee is facing the inside of your right knee. Your right knee is slightly bent and your left leg is straight. Your left hand is holding that 5-pound weight against your outer left thigh. Your foot is flexed as you bring your left leg up. When you feel that squeeze at the top, lower your leg.

Do 20 reps and get back up on your hands and knees for another stretch.

Arm-Leg Opposition Stretch

Now repeat the opposition arm-leg stretch. The rhythm is as follows: right arm, left leg, stretch and hold; left arm, right leg, stretch and hold. Repeat right arm, left leg and then left arm, right leg.

This arm-leg opposition stretch is good for your balance and will help develop spinal stabilization.

Cat Stretch

Repeat the cat stretch by rounding your back, tucking in your chin, and pulling in your abs

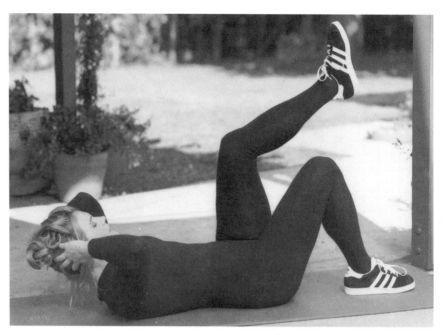

Knee-Up Crunch

as you exhale and release. Do this stretch 4 times.

Now come onto your back on the floor so we can give your abs their turn.

Crunch—Knee-Up, Knees-Up, Reverse Curl, and Three-Count Crunch

Crunch

Lie on your back with your knees bent and your hands behind your head. Support your head in your hands. Do not pull on your head or neck.

Keep your feet on the floor and lift your head and shoulders up toward your knees. Your shoulders come slightly off the floor before you return your head and shoulders back down to the floor. Your lower back remains on the floor at all times.

Do 25 reps of these crunches.

Knee-Up Crunch

Lift your right knee up so that your calf is parallel to the floor and your knee is in line with your pelvic bone. Your other foot remains on the floor, knee bent. Your head is still in your hands and your elbows are out to the side. Lift your head and shoulders off the floor. You're lifting as you exhale and pull in your abs. On the lift, aim your left shoulder toward your right (lifted) knee.

You're working your obliques here. Lower back down toward the floor and repeat.

Do 25 reps of this crunch. Then switch sides.

Lift your left knee up so that it is in line with your pelvic bone. Your right foot is flat on the floor. With your hands behind your head for support, lift your head and shoulders up off the floor and aim your right shoulder toward your left knee. Do not twist. Lift and turn slightly. Now lower.

Do 25 reps of this crunch.

Knees-Up Crunch

Bring up your other knee so that your legs form a right angle to your hips. Keep your hands behind your head and lift your head and shoulders up toward your bent knees. At the same time, pull your knees in toward your chin. Exhale as you lift. Inhale as you lower but do not touch the floor with your shoulders. Lift again.

Do 25 reps of these crunches.

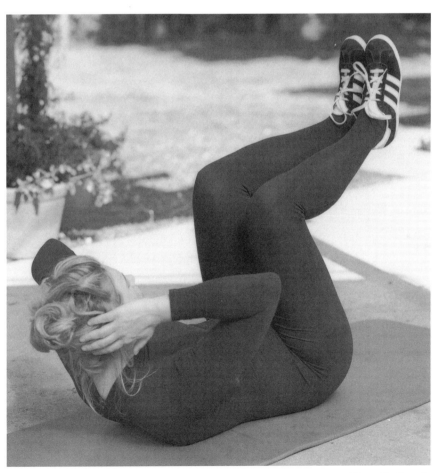

Knees-Up Crunch

Reverse Curl

Extend your legs straight up. Place your hands under your hips or right next to your hips and lift your gluts and hips up off the floor, exhaling and pulling in on your abs as you lift.

Do 25 reps.

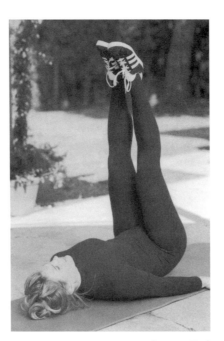

Reverse Curl

Three-Count Crunch

Bring both feet back down on the floor. Your knees are bent and your hands are behind your head. As you lift your upper body off the floor, you bring your feet up and pull your knees in toward your chin. Now bring your legs straight up as you lower your head and shoulders to the floor. Your gluts do not lift. Crunch up again by lifting your upper body and pulling in your knees as you crunch. Your hips lift a little as you pull your knees in. Now go back to the starting position with your feet on the floor and your upper body lowered to the floor but don't rest. Repeat all 3 moves.

All 3 moves equal 1 rep. Do 25 reps.

Congratulations! You've completed a superset workout. Turn to the cool-down on page 16.

We've been challenging you with our workouts as we've gone along. But it's more important that you challenge yourself, always striving for better results. After all, you can ask any actor to confirm this: If you want to look the part, you've got to act the part. Act on . . . and good luck!

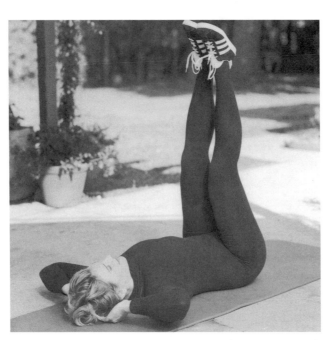

Three-Count Crunch

POSTPREGNANCY WORKOUT
MONTH 5 SUMMARY*

EXERCISE	REPS	SETS
SUPERSET 1		
Alternating Leg Lunge and Plié	10	1
SUPERSET 2		
Triceps Kick-Back		
right	15	1
left	15	1
Overhead Press	15	1
Biceps Curl	20	1
Seated Row	15	1
SUPERSET 3		
Pelvic Tilt with Bridge	10	1
Pulse	10	1
Weight on Heels	10	2
Right Leg Up/Kegel	10	1
Left Leg Up/Kegel	10	1
Pelvic Tilt	10	1

*Repeat exercises or add sets at your discretion.

EXERCISE	REPS	SETS

SUPERSET 4

Push-Up	15	1
Reverse Fly	12	1

SUPERSET 5

Side Straight-Leg Lift

right	20	1

Arm-Leg Opposition Stretch

right arm/left leg	20 count hold	1
left arm/right leg	20 count hold	1

Cat Stretch	4	1

Side Straight-Leg Lift

left	20	1

Arm-Leg Opposition Stretch

right arm/left leg	20 count hold	1
left arm/right leg	20 count hold	1

Cat Stretch	4	1

EXERCISE	REPS	SETS
SUPERSET 6		
Crunch	25	1
Knee-Up Crunch		
right	25	1
left	25	1
Knees-Up Crunch	25	1
Reverse Curl	25	1
Three-Count Crunch	25	1

Eight

A Better Primetime Body

Refining the Workout Program

We've promised you results in our five-month postpregnancy workout. We know that if you have followed our script, starting from your pregnancy days until now, you've made progress in building a better body. But Mother Nature, who sometimes seems to have her own schedule, may have dealt you a few strategically placed fat cells that you're finding very difficult to get rid of.

Don't feel singled out. You're not alone. In fact, you're in very good company. Kathy—who, you will remember, had a body composed of only 11 percent fat before she became pregnant, makes her living at keeping people in good shape, and generally does an extraordinary amount of working out in a day—was still fighting off the stubborn fat deposits on her back, upper arms, abs, and thighs six months after her babies were born.

In reaction, she created a workout that works away those last baby-fat deposits. It's not easy but it is effective. It's almost all supersets, and once again, it's the kind of workout that you can do at your convenience.

We'd like you to keep your cardio work up at four to six times a week. If you can then add our 25-minute workout, that's great. If you have to split the work up, please use our warm-up each time you work out. Your muscles need to be warmed up before you work out to avoid injury.

Our warm-up is on page 7. When you've completed the warm-up, start the following workout. Keep focused on your goal; it will help get you through the work. Good luck!

PROPS

- Straight-back chair
- Hand weights
- Rubber exercise band or panty hose

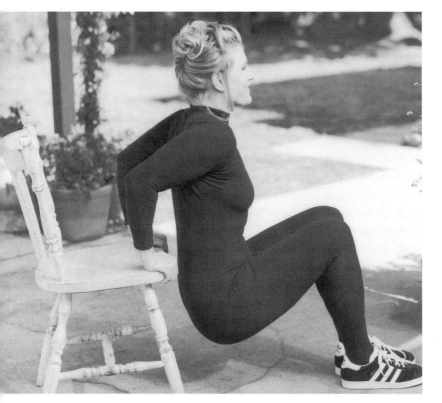

Triceps Dip

We'll start with your upper-body work. These exercises target those upper arms.

Triceps Dip

Stand with your back toward the seat of your chair. Place your hands behind you on the chair seat and bring your knees out in front of you. Lift yourself away from the chair so that your gluts and quads are level with the chair seat. With your elbows slightly bent and your fingers facing forward, dip down so that your butt and your back skim the chair as you lower. Go down only to the point where your elbows are level with your shoulders. No lower. Do not touch the floor with your butt. Inhale as you dip down and exhale as you lift up.

Do 15 reps of these dips to complete 1 set. Do 3 sets.

Triceps Kick-Back

You need both of your 3-pound weights to start.

Get into the basic standing position with your legs shoulder-width apart, knees bent, and take one weight in each hand. Bend slightly forward from the waist, and while bending your elbows, lift both arms up so that your upper arms are parallel to your back. Your forearms are parallel with the sides of your torso. Your palms are facing in toward your body.

Now, without dropping your upper arms, extend your forearms back and squeeze your triceps. Then lower your forearms. Make sure you keep your shoulders down. Exhale on the kick-back and inhale as you return down to the starting position.

Do 15 reps of these triceps kick-backs to complete 1 set. Do 3 sets.

Single-Arm Triceps Extension

Go down to the floor with your weights. Your torso is flat and your knees are bent. Your left arm is on the floor next to you. Lift your right arm, bending at your elbow. Your forearm bends back to where it is parallel to the floor and your elbow stays directly over your shoulder. Your palm and weight are facing inward.

Now lift your forearm and weight back up overhead until they are perpendicular to your body and the floor. Keep your elbow directly over your shoulder and then lower your weight again.

Do 20 reps of this single-arm extension and then switch working arms.

Rest your right arm at your side and lift your left arm, bending

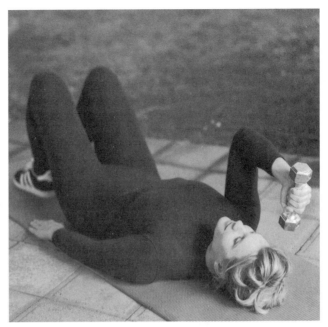

Single-Arm Triceps Extension

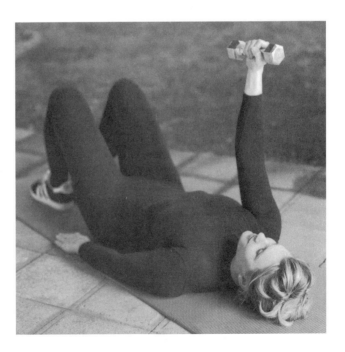

your elbow back so that your upper arm is perpendicular to your body and the floor. Your forearm bends back to where it is parallel to the floor. Your palm and weight are facing inward.

Lift your forearm and weight so they extend back up overhead. Keep your upper arm as close to your ear as possible and then lower your weight again.

Do 20 reps of this single-arm extension, then go back and repeat the entire set, doing 20 more extensions with each arm.

This next superset targets your upper back.

One-Arm Row, Reverse Fly, and Seated Row

One-Arm Row

Take your chair and place your left knee on the seat. Slightly bend your standing leg, which is your right leg. Your torso is extended forward across the seat of your chair. Your right arm is extended down from the shoulder and there is a weight in your right hand. Your palm is facing in toward your body. Your back is flat.

Now pull the weight up so that your elbow bends and comes just above your back. Now lower the weight back toward the floor.

Repeat this one-arm row for 15 reps to complete 1 set. Do 3 sets. Switch working arms.

Place your right knee on the chair seat. Your left leg is standing and your knee is slightly bent. Extend your torso forward over the seat. Your left arm is extended down from your shoulder toward the floor and your weight is facing in toward your body. Your back is flat.

Pull the weight up so that your elbow bends and comes just above your back. Lower the weight back toward the floor.

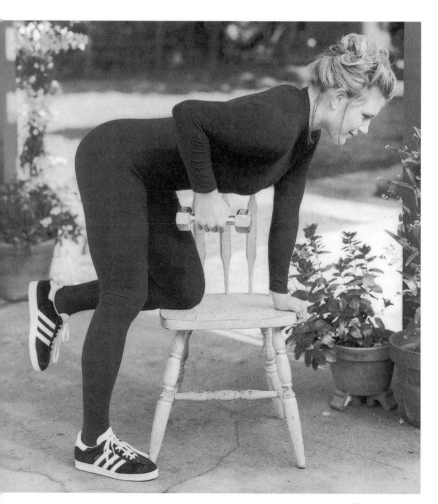

One-Arm Row

Repeat this one-arm row for 15 reps to complete 1 set. Do 3 sets.

Reverse Fly

Keep your weights and sit on the edge of your chair. Bend forward at the waist and, with a weight in each hand, lift your arms out to the sides. Bring them up to shoulder level and squeeze your shoulder blades together. Remember to keep your wrists in a neutral position and hold the weights loosely but firmly. Your head does not drop. Bring your arms back down so your knuckles are once again facing the floor. Exhale on the lift.

Do 15 reps of these reverse flys and go down to the floor with your exercise band or panty hose.

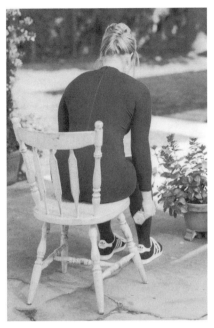

Reverse Fly

Seated Row

Sitting on the floor, extend your legs in front of you about hip-width apart. Your knees are slightly bent. Wrap the band or hose around the bottom of your flexed feet. Hold each end of the band so that your palms face inward toward your body.

Your back is straight but bent slightly forward from the waist. Pull the band backward. Your elbows bend as you pull the material while exhaling. Pull in on your abs and bring your upper

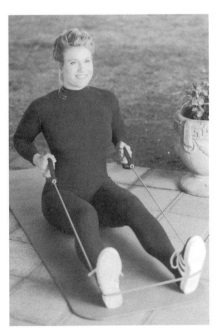

Seated Row

body into a straight position as you pull the band taut. You can feel the tension in your upper arms, shoulders, and upper back. Release your arms and keep your back straight during the repetitions.

Do 10 reps of these seated rows. Now go back and repeat the entire superset—one-arm rows, reverse flys, and seated rows—two more times.

Four-Count Crunch, Knees-In Crunch, and Nose-to-Knee

Four-Count Crunch

You're still on the floor but now you're on your back. Clasp your hands behind your head for support. Bend your knees and lift them so they are above your hips. Now lift your head and shoulders up toward your bent knees. Take your right elbow and turn it in toward your left knee, touching your left knee. Come back to center and lift your head and shoulders again; bring your upper body down but don't rest.

Do 10 reps of these four-count crunches to your left side. The counts are (1) lift center, (2) elbow to bent knee, (3) lift center, and (4) back to the beginning. Switch sides without stopping in between.

Lift your head and shoulders up toward your bent knees. Take your left elbow and turn it in toward your right knee, touching your right knee. Straighten back

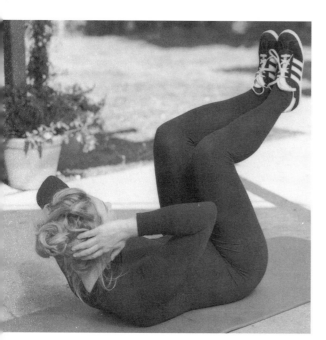

Four-Count Crunch: lift center

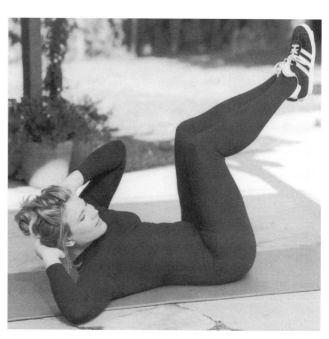

Four-Count Crunch: elbow to bent knee

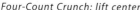

to center and lift your head and shoulders again and then come down.

Do 10 reps of these four-count crunches to your right side.

Knees-In Crunch

Stay in the same position. Your hands are cradling your head, and your knees are lifted and bent so they are over your hips. Lift your shoulders up, aim your nose toward your knees, and pull in

your abs. Come down but don't rest.

Do 15 reps of these crunches to complete 1 set. Do 3 sets.

Nose-to-Knee

Again, your knees are bent but your feet are flat on the floor. Your hands are behind your head. Now lift your upper body and aim your nose toward your bent knees. Exhale and pull in on your abs as you lift. Bring your upper body

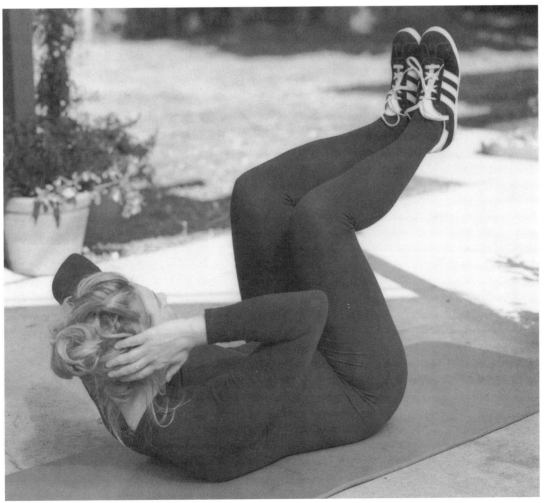

Knees-In Crunch

back down to the floor. Lift your legs straight up. Your hips come up while your upper body remains down on the floor. Now bring your legs down, by bending your knees. At the same time, lift your upper body and aim your nose toward your bent knees. Lower your feet so they tap the floor and get ready to start the four-count exercise again. Remember to exhale and pull in your abs every time you bring your upper body off the floor.

Do 15 reps of these nose-to-knee crunches to complete 1 set. Do 3 sets.

Sit-Down Squat

You can do this exercise for your gluts anywhere . . . and you can and should do them anytime. They're particularly convenient if you have a desk job. Sit on the chair seat, not too far back but not on the edge—somewhere in the middle of the seat is fine. Extend your arms straight in front of you at shoulder level. Push yourself up off the chair by pressing into your heels. As you stand, bend your elbows and pull them back so they come past your back. Bring your butt back down onto the chair seat, then extend your arms straight out again, and repeat.

Do 25 reps of these sit-down squats to complete 1 set. Do 3 sets.

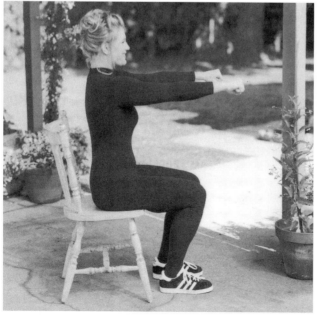
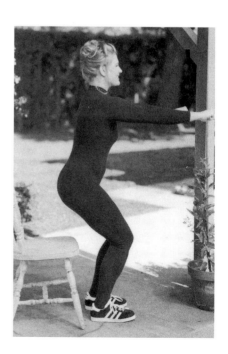

Sit-Down Squat

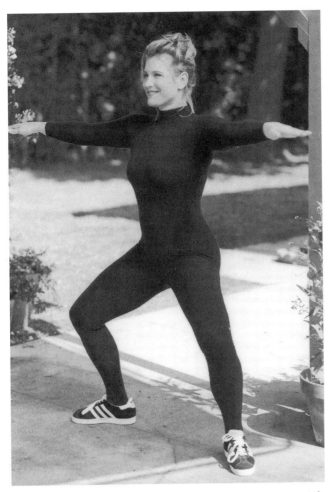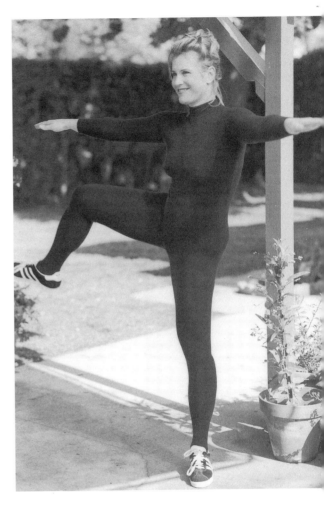

Plié with Bent Knee Lift

Plié with Bent Knee Lift/ Side Straight-Leg Lift

In your plié position, your legs are more than shoulder-width apart and your feet are on the ten o'clock and two o'clock of an imaginary clock. Your arms are extended out to the sides. Lower your torso so that your butt comes down toward the floor and your knees bend out over your toes. Do not bend beyond your toes and never go lower than knee level with your butt. Now lift and bring your right knee up toward your right elbow. Do not straighten your standing leg. Keep the knee slightly bent. Then plié again. But this time, when you come up, lift your right, straightened leg out to the side. Your right knee is facing forward and your left knee is still slightly bent. Lower your leg and plié down again. Come up while bending your right knee and

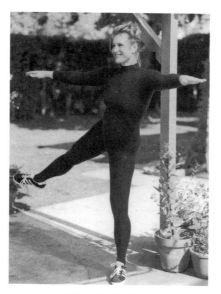

Plié with Side Straight-Leg Lift

touching your elbow with your knee.

Do 8 reps of this plié with bent right-knee lift and right-side straight-leg lift then switch working legs.

Your arms are extended out to the sides. Bend your knees and lower your torso toward the floor. Come down as far as you can but do not go lower than knee level. Lift and bring your left knee up toward your left elbow. Plié again but this time when you come up, lift your straightened left leg out

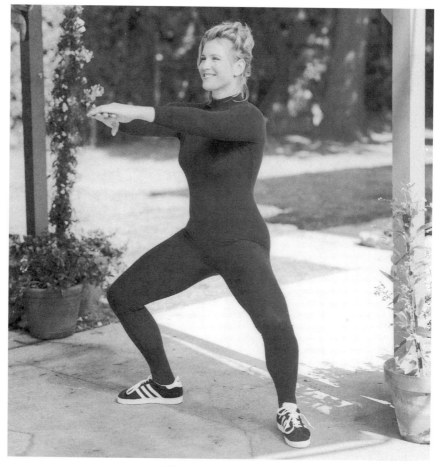

Plié with Alternating Knee Lift and Side Straight-Leg Lift

to the side. Bring this leg down into plié position and plié down. Come up and bend your left knee, reaching it toward your left elbow.

Do 8 reps of this plié with bent left-knee lift and left-side straight-leg lift.

Plié with Alternating Knee Lift/Side Straight-Leg Lift

Continue with pliés. This time you plié down, arms extended forward, knees out over toes. When you lift, pull your right knee up to the side. Bring your right leg back into starting position. Plié down, and when you lift, bring your straightened left leg out to the side. Your left knee is facing forward and your standing leg is slightly bent at the knee. Bring your left leg down into starting position. Plié and come up, bending your right knee and touching your right elbow.

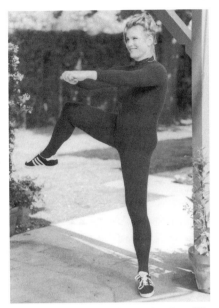

Plié with Alternating Knee Lift and Side Straight-Leg Lift

The rhythm is plié, right knee up to the side, plié, left-side straight-leg lift, which is 1 rep. Do 8 reps. Reverse.

In the plié position, lift and bend your left knee, bringing it up to the side. Lower your left leg, plié, and lift. Lift your right leg out to the side, knee facing forward. Bring your leg down to starting position and plié again.

The rhythm is plié, left knee up to the side, plié, right-side

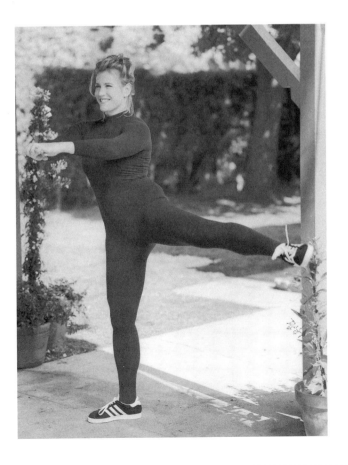

straight-leg lift, which is 1 rep. Do 8 reps.

All these pliés are giving you a cardio workout because you're using your total body weight with each move. At the same time you're working the gluteus medius, gluteus maximus, quads, and hamstrings. Time now for thighs.

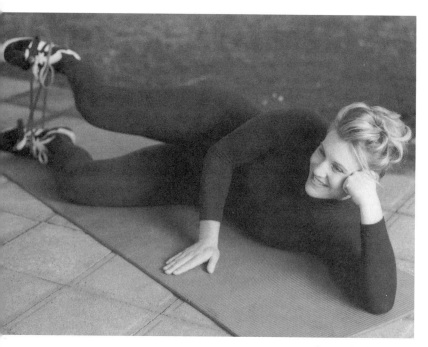

Outer-Thigh Squeeze

Outer-Thigh Squeeze

Come on down to the floor with your exercise band or panty hose. Take your band and tie the ends together so it forms a circle. Put the band around both feet so it's taut and secure. You should be on your left side, with knees bent and your head resting on your left hand. Tilt your pelvis up slightly and lift your upper leg so that you feel your outer thigh working against the resistance of the band.

Squeeze your gluts so that when you press out with your thighs, you'll work your gluts at the same time. Lower your leg and lift again.

Each squeeze up is 1 rep. Do 20 reps to complete 1 set. Do 3 sets.

Reverse sides so that you're on your right side, knees bent, with your head resting on your right hand.

Lift your left leg, using the resistance of the band to work your outer thigh muscle. Lower your leg and lift again.

Do 20 reps to complete 1 set. Do 3 sets.

Inner-Thigh Leg Lift

Come onto your left side. Extend your left arm out and rest your head on your hand. Your right arm is in front of your chest anchoring you in place. Your hips are stacked. Cross your top leg (your right leg) over your bottom leg. Bend your right knee and let your foot touch the floor in front of you. (If you have a problem keeping your hips stacked, put a pillow under your right leg.) Keep your left leg straight with your knee facing forward. Flex your left foot.

Now lift your left leg off the floor. It won't go more than an inch or two but you will work your inner thigh. Lower your leg but don't rest it. Lift it again.

Do 15 reps of these inner-thigh leg lifts to complete 1 set. Do 2 sets. Switch sides.

You're on your right side with your right arm extended out and your head resting on your right hand. Your left arm is in front of your chest. Your hips are stacked. Cross your left leg over your bottom leg. Bend your top (left) knee and keep your bottom leg straight with your knee facing forward. Flex your right foot and lift your right leg off the floor. Lower your leg but don't rest it on the bottom. Lift again.

Do 15 reps of these inner-thigh leg lifts to complete 1 set. Do 2 sets.

Come up off the floor and walk over to a mirror. Look yourself square in the eye and congratulate yourself on your performance. You're not just shaping your body, you're shaping your future. You've got the control. Your Primetime Pregnancy Workout is giving you a primetime body and a primetime attitude. You should be proud of yourself.

In fact, give yourself a hand. You deserve it.

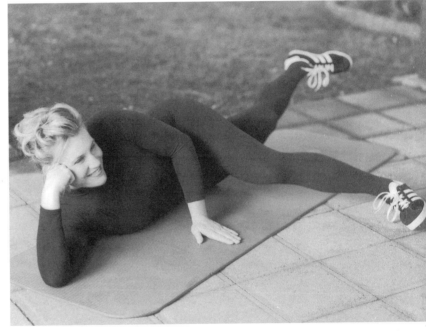

Inner-Thigh Leg Lift

A BETTER PRIMETIME BODY
THE FOLLOW-UP WORKOUT SUMMARY

EXERCISE	REPS	SETS
Triceps Dip	15	3
Triceps Kick-Back	15	3
Single-Arm Triceps Extension		
right	20	2
left	20	2

SUPERSET 1

One-Arm Row		
right	15	3
left	15	3
Reverse Fly	15	1
Seated Row	10	1

(Repeat entire superset two more times)

SUPERSET 2

Four-Count Crunch		
right	10	1
left	10	1
Knees-In Crunch	15	3
Nose-to-Knee	15	3

EXERCISE	REPS	SETS
Sit-Down Squat	25	3
Plié with Bent Knee Lift/Side Straight-Leg Lift		
right	8	1
left	8	1
Plié with Alternating KneeLift/Side Straight-Leg Lift		
right	8	1
left	8	1
Outer-Thigh Squeeze	20	3
Inner-Thigh Leg Lift		
right	15	2
left	15	2

Nine

Sorry, Wrong Number

A Primetime Message for You

If you climb on the scale at any time during our Primetime Pregnancy Workout months or at any time after and you see a number that is higher than you want, the first thing you do is step off the scale. Don't beat yourself up emotionally. Don't think that you're a failure. Don't go on an eating binge, thinking that it doesn't matter anyway.

Do evaluate your diet. Make sure you're eating lots of protein and complex carbohydrates, lots of fruits and vegetables, and very little fat. Make sure you do not eat heavy meals or skip meals. Your body needs fuel to burn fat and it needs a steady stream of fuel, not heavy loads.

Make sure you're drinking enough water: at least 64 ounces a day. Water helps pass waste through your system.

Do keep working out. Even if the pounds don't drop, the inches can drop.

Muscle weighs more than fat and muscle needs more fuel than fat so the good thing about building muscle is that you can eat more.

Don't feel alone. It happens to everybody. And everybody has to come up with her own plan to combat the pounds.

There was a point some time after her baby was born that Jami Gertz still hadn't gotten rid of her last five pounds. She thought she was doing everything right—eating right and working out diligently. Still, those pounds wouldn't drop. So she took off alone, went to a spa, and let some experts take control of her life for a few days. This sojourn gave her the opportunity to concentrate strictly on herself, and the change of routine helped her take off that extra weight.

No matter what you want, in order to get it, you've got to structure a plan and follow through. You may not be able to go to a spa but you can create a state of mind that will help you achieve your goal. It may take longer for you to get back into shape than it took Michelle Pfeiffer. It may take you less time to get back into shape than it did Kathy Kaehler. No matter how long it takes, it takes an "attitude" to keep your performance at a primetime level.

We think you've got what it takes. You should, too.

Good luck!

About the Authors

Kathy Kaehler is one of the top personal trainers in America. She is the fitness expert for the *Today* show. Her celebrity client list includes Michelle Pfeiffer, Lisa Kudrow, Jennifer Aniston, Meg Ryan, Melanie Griffith, Claudia Schiffer, Candice Bergen, Alfre Woodard, Jami Gertz, and Rita Wilson. She has starred in a number of fitness videos, including the Reebok series *Versa Training Abs and Legs* and the *Perfectly Fit* series with Claudia Schiffer. She is the proud mother of twins Payton and Cooper Koch.

Cynthia Tivers is a Hollywood writer, producer, and director. Among her many television credits are *Good Morning America*, *Lifestyles of the Rich and Famous*, and *Showtime* feature programs. She has produced various talk and magazine shows, specials, and documentaries. She has written for a number of national magazines, including *Fitness*, *Woman's Day*, and *Ladies' Home Journal*, and she is the author of *World Class Legs*, a Book-of-the-Month Club selection. She has also written home-exercise videos for supermodels Kathy Ireland and Rachel Hunter.

Kathy and Cynthia coauthored the exercise book *Primetime Bodies*, which was a Book-of-the-Month Club selection.